APPLIED ECONOMETRICS FOR HEALTH ECONOMISTS – A PRACTICAL GUIDE

Andrew M Jones

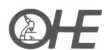

Office of Health Economics
12 Whitehall London SW1A 2DY
www.ohe.org

© December 2001. Office of Health Economics. Price £10.00

ISBN 1 899040 17 X

Printed by BSC Print Ltd, London.

About the author

Andrew Jones is Professor of Economics at the University of York, where he directs the graduate programme in health economics. He researches and publishes extensively in the area of microeconometrics and health economics. Andrew is an organiser of European workshops on econometrics and health economics; joint editor, *Health Economics;* joint editor, *Health Economics Letters;* and associate editor, *Journal of Health Economics.*

OFFICE OF HEALTH ECONOMICS

Terms of Reference

The Office of Health Economics (OHE) was founded in 1962. Its terms of reference are to:

- commission and undertake research on the economics of health and health care;

- collect and analyse health and health care data from the UK and other countries;

- disseminate the results of this work and stimulate discussion of them and their policy implications.

The OHE is supported by an annual grant from the Association of the British Pharmaceutical Industry, by income for commissioned research and consultancy, and by sales of its publications.

Independence

The research and editorial independence of the OHE is ensured by its Policy Board:

Peer Review

All OHE publications have been reviewed by members of its Editorial Board and, where appropriate, other clinical or technical experts independent of the authors. The current membership of the Editorial Board is as follows:

CONTENTS

1 Introduction

1.1 Overview

Given the extensive use of individual-level survey data in health economics, it is increasingly important to understand the econometric techniques available to applied researchers. Moreover, it is just as important to be aware of the limitations and pitfalls associated with each technique. The purpose of this booklet is to introduce readers to the appropriate econometric techniques for use with different forms of survey data – known collectively as microeconometrics. There is a strong emphasis on applied work, illustrating the use of relevant computer software applied to large-scale survey data sets. The aim is to illustrate the steps involved in doing microeconometric research:

- formulate empirical problems involving large survey data sets;
- select an appropriate econometric method;
- be aware of the methods of estimation that are available for qualitative and limited dependent variables and the software that can be used to implement them;
- construct usable data sets and know the limitations of survey design;
- interpret the results of the analysis in a meaningful way.

The standard linear regression model familiar from econometric textbooks is designed to deal with a dependent variable (y) which varies continuously over a range between minus infinity and plus infinity. Unfortunately this standard model is rarely applicable with survey data, where qualitative and categorical variables are more common. This booklet therefore deals with practical analysis of qualitative and categorical variables. The booklet assumes basic familiarity with the principles of statistical inference – estimation and hypothesis testing – and with the linear regression model. An accessible and clear overview of the linear regression model is given in Peter Kennedy's *A Guide to Econometrics* published by the MIT Press and the material is covered in many other introductory econometrics textbooks.

Technical details or derivations are avoided and the booklet concentrates on the intuition behind the models and their interpretation. Key terms are marked in **bold** and defined in the **Glossary**. Formulas are presented in the **Technical Appendix**. The **References** are augmented with a list of further **Suggested Further**

Reading for those who would like to pursue the topics in more detail. All of the results presented have been estimated using Stata Version 7 and the **Stata Code Appendix** lists the Stata commands that were used. To give a feel for the way that the software package presents results the tables are reproduced as they appear in the Stata output. The text only refers to key results and readers who want a full explanation of all of the statistics listed are encouraged to consult the Stata user manuals.

1.2 Identification and estimation

The evaluation problem is whether it is possible to identify causal effects from empirical data. An understanding of the implications of the evaluation problem for statistical analysis will help to provide a motivation for many of the econometric methods discussed below.

Consider an *outcome* y_{it}, for individual i at time t; for example an individual's level of use of health care services. The problem is to identify the effect of a *treatment*, for example whether the individual has purchased health insurance, on the outcome. The causal effect of interest is the difference between the outcome with the treatment and the outcome without the treatment. But this *pure causal effect* cannot be identified from empirical data. This is because the *counterfactual* can never be observed. The basic problem is that the individual 'cannot be in two places at the same time'; that is we cannot observe their use of health care, at time t, both with and without the influence of insurance.

One response to this problem is to concentrate on the *average causal effect* and attempt to estimate it with sample data by comparing the average outcome among those receiving the treatment with the average outcome among those who do not receive the treatment. The problem for statistical inference arises if there are unobserved factors that influence both whether an individual is selected into the treatment group and also how they respond to the treatment. This will lead to biased estimates of the treatment effect. For example, someone who knows they have a high risk of illness may be more prone to take out health insurance and they will also tend to use more health care. Unless the analyst is able to control for their level of risk, this will lead to spurious evidence of a positive relationship between having health insurance and using health care.

A randomised experimental design may be able to control for this bias and, in some circumstances, a natural experiment may mimic the features of a controlled experiment. However, the vast majority of econometric studies rely on observational data gathered in a non-experimental setting. In the absence of experimental data attention has to focus on alternative estimation strategies:

- **instrumental variables (IV)** – variables (or 'instruments') that are good predictors of the treatment, but are not independently related to the outcome, may be used to purge the bias. In practice the validity of the IV approach relies on finding appropriate instruments and these may be hard to find (see Jones, 2000, for further discussion);

- corrections for selection bias – these range from parametric methods such as the **Heckit** estimator to more recent **semiparametric** estimators. The use of these techniques in health economics is discussed in Section 7;
- longitudinal data – the availability of **panel data**, giving repeated measurements for a particular individual, provides the opportunity to control for unobservable individual effects which remain constant over time. Panel data models are discussed in Section 10.

So far, the discussion has concentrated on the evaluation problem. More generally, most econometric work in health economics focuses on the problem of finding an appropriate model to fit the available data. *Classical linear regression analysis* assumes that the relationship between an outcome, or dependent variable, y, and the explanatory, or independent, variables, X, can be summarised by a regression function. The regression function is a linear function of the X variables and of a random error term, ϵ. This relationship can be written using the following shorthand notation:

$$y = X\beta + \epsilon \qquad (1)$$

The random error term ϵ captures all of the variation in y that is not explained by the X variables. The classical model assumes that this error term:

- has a mean of zero;
- that its variance, σ^2, is the same across all the observations (this is known as **homoscedasticity**);
- that values of the error term are independent across observations (known as serial independence);
- that values of the error term are independent of the values of the X variables.

Often it is assumed that the error term has a **normal distribution**.

In health economics, empirical analysis is complicated by the fact that the theoretical models often involve inherently unobservable (latent) concepts such as health endowments, agency and supplier inducement, or quality of life. The widespread use of individual level survey data means that nonlinear models are common in health economics. Examples of these nonlinear models include:

- binary responses, such as whether the individual has visited their doctor over the previous month (see Section 3);
- multinomial responses, such as the choice of health care provider (see Sections 4 and 5); integer counts, such as the number of visits to a doctor per time period (see Section 8);
- measures of duration, such as the time elapsed between visits (see Section 9).

Throughout the rest of the text, emphasis is placed on the assumptions underpinning these econometric models and applied empirical examples are provided. The empirical examples are based on a single data set, the Health and Lifestyle Survey (HALS). The next section describes how the survey was collected and the kind of information it contains.

2 The Health and Lifestyle Survey

The Health and Lifestyle Survey (HALS) was designed as a representative survey of adults in Great Britain (see Cox et al., 1987; 1993). The population surveyed was individuals aged 18 and over living in private households. In principle, each individual should have an equal probability of being selected for the survey. This allows the data to be used to make inferences about the underlying population. HALS was designed as a **cross-section survey** with one measurement for each observation, or individual. It was carried out between the Autumn of 1984 and the Summer of 1985. Information was collected in three stages:

- a one-hour face-to-face interview, which collected information on experience and attitudes towards health and lifestyle along with general socio-economic information;
- a nurse visit to collect physiological measures and indicators of cognitive function, such as memory and reasoning;
- a self-completion postal questionnaire to measure psychiatric health and personality.

The HALS is an example of a clustered random sample. The intention was to build a representative random sample of this population. Addresses were randomly selected from electoral registers using a three-stage design. First 198 electoral constituencies were selected with the probability of selection proportional to the population of each constituency. Then two wards were selected for each constituency and, finally, 30 addresses per ward. Individuals were randomly selected from households. This selection procedure gave a target of 12,672 interviews.

Of the addresses from the electoral register, 418 proved to be inappropriate as they were in use as holiday homes, business premises or were derelict. This left a total of 12,254 individuals to be interviewed. The response rate fell more dramatically when it came to success in completing these interviews: 9,003 interviews were completed. This is a response rate of 73.5%. In other words, there was a one in four chance that an interview was not completed. The missing values are an example of **unit non-response**. For these individuals, no information is available from any of the survey questions. The main reason for non-response is refusal on the part of the interviewee or their family. This accounted for 2,341 cases or 19%

of the requests for interview. Further cases were lost because the interviewer was unable to establish contact or for other reasons, such as illness or incapacity on the part of the interviewee.

A question for researchers is whether the 1 in 4 individuals who were not included in the survey are systematically different from those who did respond. If there are systematic differences, this creates a problem of **sample selection bias** and it will not be possible to claim that inferences based on the observed data are representative of the underlying population. What do we know about the people who did not participate in the interview? Although the survey provides no information, we do know the addresses of the non-responders. This allows us to compare response rates across geographic areas and to use other sources of information about those areas. For example, analysis of the HALS data shows that response rates were particularly low in Greater London with a response rate of 64.2% compared to 73.5% on average. The representativeness of the sample can be gauged further by comparing the observed data with external data sources. So, for example, the HALS team compared their survey to the 1981 census. This comparison suggests that the HALS data under-represent men and over-represent women with only 43.3% of men amongst the interviewees compared with 47.7% in the census.

The overall response rate of 73.5% is fairly typical of general population surveys. Understandably, the response rate declines for the subsequent nurse visit and postal questionnaire. The overall response rate for individuals who completed all three stages of the survey is only 53.7%. Comparison with the 1981 census suggests that this final sample under-represents those with lower incomes and lower levels of education. It is important to bear unit non-response in mind when analysing any survey data sets.

The HALS data were originally intended to be a one-off cross-section survey and most of the examples used in this booklet are drawn from the original cross-section. However, HALS also provides an example of a longitudinal or **panel data** set. In 1991/92, seven years on from the original survey, the HALS was repeated. This provides an example of repeated measurements where the same individuals are re-interviewed. Panel data provide a powerful enhancement of cross-section surveys that allows a deeper analysis of heterogeneity across individuals and of changes in individual behaviour over time. However, because of the need to revisit and interview individuals repeatedly, the problems of unit non-response tend to be amplified. Of the original 9,003 individuals who were interviewed at the time of the first HALS survey 808 (9%) had died by the time of the second survey, 1,347 (14.9%) could not be traced and 222 were traced but could not be interviewed, either because they had moved overseas or they had moved to geographic areas that were out of the scope of the survey. These cases are examples of attrition – individuals who drop out of a longitudinal survey. Systematic differences between the individuals who stay in and those who drop out can lead to **attrition bias**.

A further source of missing data is **item non-response**. This occurs when an individual responds to the interview as a whole but is unwilling or unable to answer a particular question. Non-responses are coded as 'missing values' in the dataset. Again researchers should be aware of the potential bias this creates if observations with missing values are systematically different from those who respond to the question. For example, the self-employed may be less willing to reveal information about their income than those in paid employment.

3 Binary Dependent Variables

3.1 Methods

It is often the case in survey data that the outcome of interest is measured as a **binary variable**, taking values of either one or zero. Often this binary variable will indicate whether an individual is a participant or a non-participant. Examples include: health care utilisation, such as whether an individual has visited a doctor in the previous month or whether they have used prescription drugs; or whether a household has purchased health insurance; or whether an individual is a current smoker. If the binary outcome y, depends on a set of explanatory variables X, then the conditional expectation of y given X, in other words the average value of y that individuals with characteristics X are likely to report, is equal to the probability that y = 1, that is:

$$E(y| X) = P(y=1| X) = F(X) \tag{2}$$

A simple way to model binary data is to use a linear function, for which we can use the shorthand notation $F(X) = X\beta$. This gives the **linear probability model**. The linear probability model is straightforward to estimate, using standard software for the method of **ordinary least squares.**

These estimates should be adjusted for the fact that, by design, the error term in the equation cannot have a normal distribution. Normality implies that the error is continuous and can take any value between plus and minus infinity. In the linear probability model, the error term can take only two values corresponding to values of zero or one for the dependent variable. The variance of this implied error term depends on the value of the X's. In other words, by design, the error term is **heteroscedastic** (meaning that it varies across individuals with different values of X). This can be corrected by using **weighted least squares**, rather than ordinary least squares.

In practice, the linear probability model may provide a reasonable approximation for binary choice models, so long as the function F(.) is approximately linear over the range of sample observations. But a major drawback of the method is that, because a straight line is used, predicted values of the regression function can lie outside the range zero to one. Equation (2) shows that these predicted values correspond to the probability that an individual participates. This means that the linear probability model can lead to logical inconsistencies, with predicted probabilities outside the logical range zero to one. A way to avoid this is to use a non-linear function for F(.). Popular choices are 'S' curves, that are bounded to the range [0,1] whatever the values of the regressors X. The most common choices of these 'S' curves are **logit** and **probit** models.

Logit and probit models are often motivated in terms of a latent variable specification. This assumes that there is some continuous latent variable y^* that determines participation. You can think of y^* as an individual's propensity to participate. If y^* is positive, the individual will choose to participate and the observed binary outcome equals 1. Otherwise, the individual will not participate and the observed value equals 0. Then the latent variable y^* is modelled by a linear regression function of the individual characteristics X. Assuming that the error term in this equation has a standard normal distribution gives the probit model. Assuming that it has a standard **logistic distribution** gives the logit model. The probability functions for the probit and logit models both have the characteristic S shape and are similar in appearance, although the logit model gives more weight to the tails of the distribution. As with many of the models described in this booklet, logit and probit models are typically estimated by the method of **maximum likelihood estimation**.

TABLE 1 - LINEAR PROBABILITY MODEL OF SAH (WLS)

Source	SS	df	MS		
Model	71.8679703	27	2.66177668		
Residual	1813.16391	8867	.204484483		
Total	1885.03188	8894	.211944219		

Number of obs = 8895
F(27, 8867) = 13.02
Prob > F = 0.0000
R-squared = 0.0381
Adj R-squared = 0.0352
Root MSE = .4522

yvar	Coef.	Std. Err.	t	P>|t|	[95% Conf. Interval]	
male	.0110496	.0116204	0.95	0.342	-.0117291	.0338283
age	-.0028952	.0007957	-3.64	0.000	-.0044549	-.0013354
age2	-.0107486	.0028589	-3.76	0.000	-.0163527	-.0051444
age3	.0404218	.0095455	4.23	0.000	.0217105	.0591331
ethbawi	-.1076602	.0435029	-2.47	0.013	-.1929359	-.0223845
ethipb	-.0876126	.038631	-2.27	0.023	-.1633383	-.0118869
ethothnw	-.1256814	.0542635	-2.32	0.021	-.2320504	-.0193124
part	.0644476	.018349	3.51	0.000	.0284793	.100416
unemp	-.0445345	.021623	-2.06	0.039	-.0869206	-.0021485
retd	.0193786	.0209592	0.92	0.355	-.0217062	.0604634
stdnt	.072331	.0536686	1.35	0.178	-.0328719	.177534
keephse	-.0292059	.0168368	-1.73	0.083	-.0622098	.003798
lsch14u	-.0743648	.0281281	-2.64	0.008	-.1295023	-.0192273
lsch14	-.075411	.0178249	-4.23	0.000	-.1103518	-.0404701
lsch15	-.0407599	.0147827	-2.76	0.006	-.0697375	-.0117823
lsch17	.0146558	.020515	0.71	0.475	-.0255583	.05487
lsch18	.0798895	.0233398	3.42	0.001	.0341381	.1256409
lsch19	.0114685	.0454503	0.25	0.801	-.0776246	.1005616
regsc1s	.0966774	.0272621	3.55	0.000	.0432373	.1501174
regsc2	.0772081	.0144526	5.34	0.000	.0488776	.1055385
regsc3n	.0351518	.0155857	2.26	0.024	.0046003	.0657033
regsc4	-.0281103	.0135481	-2.07	0.038	-.0546678	-.0015528
regsc5n	-.0674235	.0195772	-3.44	0.001	-.1057993	-.0290476
widow	-.0556353	.0185643	-3.00	0.003	-.0920257	-.0192449
single	-.0309911	.0166773	-1.86	0.063	-.0636824	.0017002
seprd	-.097271	.0311903	-3.12	0.002	-.1584112	-.0361309
divorce	-.0648466	.0243986	-2.66	0.008	-.1126735	-.0170196
_cons	.7544911	.0179991	41.92	0.000	.7192087	.7897735

RESET test;

F(1, 8866) = 4.42
Prob > F = 0.0355

3.2 Results for the linear probability model

To illustrate the estimation and interpretation of linear probability, logit and probit models, we will use HALS data on individuals' self-assessed health (SAH). In HALS, self-assessed health is measured on a four-point scale with categories 'excellent', 'good', 'fair' and 'poor'. To illustrate binary choice models, this is collapsed into a binary variable where y = 1, if an individual reports excellent or good health, and y = 0, if an individual reports fair or poor health. The aim is to model the probability of an individual reporting excellent or good health as a function of a range of socio-economic characteristics, including the individual's gender, age, ethnic origin, work status, educational qualifications, occupational socio-economic group and marital status.

Table 1 presents the **weighted least squares (WLS)** estimates for a linear probability model based on a variety of explanatory variables. The variables include the individual's sex, age, ethnic origin, employment status, the age at which they left school, social class and marital status. The WLS estimates are computed in two steps. First, the model is estimated using **ordinary least squares** and the predicted values from this equation are saved. These predictions are then used to calculate weights. This is possible only if the predictions lie within the range [0,1]. So, any logically inconsistent predictions mean that it is not possible to use weighted least squares. In the example reported here, this was not a problem as all of the predictions are in the required range.

One attraction of the linear probability model is its ease of interpretation. As we have seen in (1), the regression function, E(y|X), can be interpreted as the probability of participating given the values of X, and here this is assumed to be a linear function. This means that the regression coefficients ß are measured in units of probability. So, for example, consider the constant term 0.754 (in the final row of Table 1). This is the value of the regression function when all of the X variables equal 0. You can think of this as a 'reference individual'. In this example, the X variables have been constructed so that the reference individual is a woman aged 45 who is white, in full-time employment, left school at 16, is in a skilled manual occupation and is married. The coefficient tells us that this type of individual has a probability of 0.754 of reporting excellent or good health, rather than fair or poor health.

The coefficients on the X variables tell us how this probability changes with changes in the individual's characteristics. The regression function includes two types of explanatory variable. The first type can be treated as though they were **continuous variables**. The example here is the individual's age measured in years. All of the other explanatory variables are **binary** or **dummy variables**. These take the value 1 if the individual has a particular characteristic, for example if they are unemployed, and 0 otherwise. For continuous explanatory variables, we look at the impact of a small change in the variable on the probability of participation. This is known as the **marginal effect**. Here we could look at the impact of age on the probability of reporting excellent or good health. For the dummy variables, it does not make sense to think in terms of small changes. An individual either has a characteristic or does not. Here, we look at the **average effect**, for example the difference in the probability of reporting excellent or good health if someone is unemployed compared to someone who is employed.

An attraction of the linear probability model is that the regression coefficients directly measure both the marginal effects of the continuous explanatory variables and the average effects of the dummy explanatory variables.

The *sign* of the coefficients tells us about the **qualitative effect** of the explanatory variables. For example, Table 1 shows that the coefficient on unemployment (unemp) is negative (–0.045). This means that an individual who is currently unemployed has a lower probability of reporting good or excellent health relative to the reference individual who is employed. The size of the coefficient tells us about the **quantitative effect** of the variable. The coefficient on unemployment is –0.045. This is measured in units of probability and tells us that the probability of reporting good or excellent health is 0.045 lower for someone who is unemployed than for the reference individual.

We are relying on a **point estimate** (–0.045) of the impact of unemployment. The fact that this estimate is different from zero may simply be due to chance, attributable to sampling variability. This sampling variability is summarised by the standard error of the coefficient. The null hypothesis that the coefficient equals zero can be tested by looking at the t-ratio; given by the ratio of the coefficient to its standard error. t-ratios are reported in the fourth column of Table 1 and the corresponding p-value (the implied significance level of the test) is given in the fifth column. With a t-ratio of –2.06, and hence a p-value of 0.039, we can say that the coefficient on unemployment is statistically significant at conventional levels of significance.

Now consider the other variables included in the model. The qualitative effects for occupational socio-economic group show that those in social classes 1, 2 and 3 (non-manual) have positive coefficients (regsc1s, regsc2, regsc3n). In other words, they are more likely to report good or excellent health compared to the reference individual who is in social class 3 – skilled manual occupations. Individuals in social classes 4 and 5 – semi-skilled and unskilled occupations – have negative coefficients (regsc4, regsc5n), showing that, on average, they are less likely than the reference individual to report good or excellent health. The quantitative effects show some evidence of a gradient in health across socio-economic groups.

A similar pattern emerges for education. Here, the reference category is leaving school at age 16. The qualitative effects show that those who left school at 15, 14 or under (lsch15, lsch14, lsch14u) are less likely to report good or excellent health, while those who left school at 17 or older (lsch17, lsch18, lsch19) are more likely to report good or excellent health.

A further note of caution is that the coefficients on the explanatory variables tell us about the impact of changing each variable when *holding all of the others constant*. This means that the age variables need to be interpreted with care because the model also includes the square and the cube of age. The fact that the level of age has a negative coefficient does not mean anything in itself. In other words, it is not possible to increase age by one year without also changing the values of age-squared and age-cubed. To understand how self-assessed health changes with age, you would need to look simultaneously at the change in all three variables.

The interpretation of the results so far assumes that the model we are using is well-specified. For example, choosing the **probit model** assumes that the function F(.) is the normal distribution function and that its argument is linear in the X variables. This may not be the case. A convenient way of testing the specification of the model is to use a regression error specification test **(RESET)**. This is a general test for problems with the assumed functional form of the model and with omitted variables – other explanatory variables that have not been included in the model and are correlated both with the dependent variable and with the included explanatory variables.

The RESET test is easy to implement. It involves saving the predicted values from the regression function, taking the squares of those values and re-estimating the model with this new variable added as an extra explanatory variable. If the model is well specified this new test variable should not be significant. If the model is poorly specified the test variable will be significant. A convenient way of carrying out the test is to look at either the t-ratio or the F test for the null hypothesis that the coefficient on the new variable equals zero (note that the t-ratio squared equals the F test). For the linear probability model of self-assessed health, reported in Table 1, the RESET test gives an F test statistic of 4.42 (p = 0.036). Although this passes a conventional 5% significance test, the size of the statistic may be a cause for a concern.

```
Probit estimates                                Number of obs   =      8895
                                                LR chi2(27)     =    401.12
                                                Prob > chi2     =    0.0000
Log likelihood = -5116.0659                     Pseudo R2       =    0.0377

------------------------------------------------------------------------------
      yvar |      Coef.   Std. Err.       z    P>|z|     [95% Conf. Interval]
-------------+----------------------------------------------------------------
      male |   .0259246   .0349187      0.74   0.458    -.0425147     .094364
       age |  -.0090254   .0023664     -3.81   0.000    -.0136634    -.0043873
      age2 |  -.0367239   .0085666     -4.29   0.000    -.0535141    -.0199338
      age3 |   .1365391    .028456      4.80   0.000     .0807664     .1923118
   ethbawi |  -.3066757   .1349111     -2.27   0.023    -.5710966    -.0422549
    ethipb |  -.2609027   .1178873     -2.21   0.027    -.4919575    -.0298479
   ethothnw |  -.3625705   .1654855     -2.19   0.028    -.6869162    -.0382248
      part |   .1652719   .0535621      3.09   0.002     .0602922     .2702517
     unemp |  -.1370677   .0661254     -2.07   0.038     -.266671    -.0074643
      retd |   .0361686   .0635569      0.57   0.569    -.0884006     .1607378
     stdnt |   .1221332   .1516553      0.81   0.421    -.1751057     .4193722
    keephse |  -.0800694   .0506691     -1.58   0.114     -.179379     .0192402
    lsch14u |  -.2164274    .085988     -2.52   0.012    -.3849608     -.047894
     lsch14 |  -.2203339   .0532942     -4.13   0.000    -.3247886    -.1158793
     lsch15 |  -.1453882   .0437683     -3.32   0.001    -.2311724    -.0596039
     lsch17 |   .0544842   .0597137      0.91   0.362    -.0625526     .1715209
     lsch18 |   .2686861   .0650129      4.13   0.000     .1412631     .3961091
     lsch19 |  -.0170855   .1317568     -0.13   0.897    -.2753242     .2411531
    regscls |    .286181   .0766413      3.73   0.000     .1359668     .4363951
     regsc2 |   .2349733   .0424138      5.54   0.000     .1518438     .3181028
    regsc3n |   .1022324   .0465856      2.19   0.028     .0109263     .1935386
     regsc4 |  -.0698505    .041477     -1.68   0.092    -.1511439     .0114429
    regsc5n |  -.1915523   .0604116     -3.17   0.002    -.3099569    -.0731477
     widow |  -.1507873   .0571748     -2.64   0.008    -.2628478    -.0387269
    single |  -.0850688    .049903     -1.70   0.088    -.1828769     .0127393
     seprd |  -.2498267   .0966871     -2.58   0.010      -.43933    -.0603233
    divorce |  -.2015977   .0743637     -2.71   0.007    -.3473478    -.0558476
     _cons |   .7248271   .0536818     13.50   0.000     .6196127     .8300416
------------------------------------------------------------------------------
```

3.3 Results for the probit model

How do the results for the linear probability model compare to those for the probit and logit models? Table 2 shows the estimates for the probit model, computed using the method of maximum likelihood estimation. Like the linear probability model, the table includes coefficients, their standard errors and z-ratios. The z-ratio is computed in the same way as the t-ratio, by taking the ratio of the coefficient and the standard error. Hypothesis testing in models estimated by maximum likelihood has to rely on the sample size being large enough for the coefficients to follow a normal distribution (a so-called **asymptotic** property). With a large sample size the z-ratio has a standard normal distribution.

The interpretation of the probit coefficients is different from the linear probability model. Recall that the probit model takes a linear function of the explanatory variables and applies a non-linear transformation, in this case using the S-curve of the normal distribution function. The coefficients relate to the underlying linear index. These are often interpreted in terms of the latent variable y^*. But y^* is by definition unobservable and is not measured in any kind of natural units, unlike the probability of participation. In themselves, the coefficients should therefore be interpreted only as qualitative effects.

So, for example, a negative coefficient means that somebody is less likely to be a participant, and a positive coefficient means they are more likely to be a participant. Unemployment (unemp) has a coefficient of –0.137 in the probit model. This cannot be compared directly with the coefficient from the linear probability model. The qualitative interpretation is that, due to the negative coefficient, the unemployed are less likely to report good or excellent health. Similarly, the qualitative results show that those in professional and managerial occupations (regsc1s, regsc2) are more likely to report good or excellent health, while those in semi-skilled and unskilled occupations (regsc4, regsc5n) are less likely to report good or excellent health. Also, those with more education (lsch17, lsch18) are more likely to report good health (with the possible exception of those who left school at age 19 or more – lsch19) and those with fewer years of education are less likely to.

TABLE 3 — AVERAGE AND MARGINAL EFFECTS FOR PROBIT MODEL

```
Probit estimates                                    Number of obs =    8895
                                                    LR chi2(27)   =  401.12
                                                    Prob > chi2   =  0.0000
Log likelihood = -5116.0659                         Pseudo R2     =  0.0377
```

yvar	dF/dx	Std. Err.	z	P>|z|	x-bar	[95% C.I.]
male*	.0086665	.0116609	0.74	0.458	.434401	-.014188 .031521
age	-.0030203	.0007916	-3.81	0.000	.83946	-.004572 -.001469
age2	-.0122893	.002865	-4.29	0.000	3.13702	-.017905 -.006674
age3	.0456916	.0095162	4.80	0.000	.242169	.02704 .064343
ethbawi*	-.1105744	.0515425	-2.27	0.023	.010455	-.211596 -.009553
ethipb*	-.0931605	.0443748	-2.21	0.027	.01439	-.180133 -.006187
ethothnw*	-.1321513	.0641797	-2.19	0.028	.007307	-.257941 -.006361
part*	.0531546	.0164963	3.09	0.002	.121529	.020822 .085487
unemp*	-.0474578	.0236162	-2.07	0.038	.05059	-.093745 -.001171
retd*	.0120303	.0210101	0.57	0.569	.221248	-.029149 .053209
stdnt*	.0393671	.0469502	0.81	0.421	.011804	-.052654 .131388
keephse*	-.0272401	.0175111	-1.58	0.114	.139966	-.061561 .007081
lsch14u*	-.0763619	.0317401	-2.52	0.012	.036875	-.138571 -.014153
lsch14*	-.0759303	.018846	-4.13	0.000	.252839	-.112868 -.038993
lsch15*	-.0495614	.0151727	-3.32	0.001	.271951	-.079299 -.019823
lsch17*	.017986	.0194367	0.91	0.362	.088477	-.020109 .056081
lsch18*	.0835677	.0185724	4.13	0.000	.088477	.047167 .119969
lsch19*	-.0057455	.0445217	-0.13	0.897	.013491	-.093006 .081515
regsc1s*	.0879753	.0213358	3.73	0.000	.056886	.046158 .129793
regsc2*	.0754063	.0129869	5.54	0.000	.223834	.049952 .10086
regsc3n*	.0334431	.0148789	2.19	0.028	.140866	.004281 .062605
regsc4*	-.0236895	.0142495	-1.68	0.092	.167285	-.051618 .004239
regsc5n*	-.0670684	.0220073	-3.17	0.002	.060371	-.110202 -.023935
widow*	-.0522256	.0204307	-2.64	0.008	.085779	-.092269 -.012182
single*	-.0289269	.0172294	-1.70	0.088	.17077	-.062696 .004842
seprd*	-.0889232	.0362115	-2.58	0.010	.021585	-.159897 -.01795
divorce*	-.0708975	.0272959	-2.71	0.007	.037549	-.124396 -.017399

```
obs. P |   .714896
pred. P |  .7233723  (at x-bar)
```

(*) dF/dx is for discrete change of dummy variable from 0 to 1
    z and P>|z| are the test of the underlying coefficient being 0

```
. * RESET test;
chi2( 1) =    0.27
        Prob > chi2 =    0.6031
```

Average and marginal effects

In order to interpret the quantitative implications of the results, we need to compute marginal effects for the continuous explanatory variables and average effects for the binary explanatory variables. Unlike the linear probability model, the marginal or average effects are not given by the coefficients directly but they can be computed from them. The formula for the **marginal effect** of an explanatory variable X_k is:

$$\partial P(y=1|X)/\partial X_k = \beta_k f(X\beta) \qquad (3)$$

where $f(.) = \partial F(.)/\partial(X\beta)$. The formula for the **average effect** of a binary variable is:

$$P(y=1| X_k =1) - P(y=1| X_k =0) = F(X\beta| X_k =1) - F(X\beta| X_k =0) \qquad (4)$$

These are more complex formulas than the linear probability model due to the non-linearity of the $F(.)$ curve. Also, it should be clear that both the marginal and average effects depend on the values of the X variables. In other words, they are different for different types of individual. The size of the effect of a variable, say unemployment, will depend on the value of the other explanatory variables, such as education, marital status and age. The common way of dealing with this is to evaluate the effect at the sample mean of the other X variables, treating this as a 'typical' observation. This is the approach adopted in software packages such as Limdep and Stata. However, this can be a rather artificial approach, especially when the Xs include dummy variables, as the typical observation is unlikely to correspond to any actual observation. An alternative is to compute the effect for each observation, using their specific X-values, and then report summary statistics at the sample mean of the effects.

Table 3 presents the average and marginal effects for the probit model as computed automatically by the *dprobit* command in Stata. The effects in Table 3 can be given a quantitative interpretation and are measured in units of probability. Consider the impact of unemployment. Here the average effect is −0.047, which is very similar to the estimate of −0.045 of the linear probability model (see Table 1). It tells us that on average the probability of an unemployed individual reporting good or excellent health is 0.047 less than for the reference individual. In this case, the estimated effect of unemployment is quite similar across the linear probability and probit specifications. However, comparing the estimates for other explanatory variables shows that this is not always the case. For example, the average effect of being in part-time (part), rather than full-time, work is 0.053 in the probit model (Table 3) compared with 0.064 in the linear probability model (Table 1).

Finally, Table 3 presents the RESET test for the probit model. As the probit model is estimated by maximum likelihood, an appropriate way of testing the null hypothesis that the coefficient on the new variables equals zero is to use a chi-squared test. The chi-squared test is calculated as twice the difference between the log-likelihood of the unrestricted model and the log-likelihood of the restricted model in which the coefficient is constrained to equal zero. Unlike the linear probability model, there is no evidence of mis-specification and the chi-squared test statistic is 0.27 with a p-value well above conventional significance levels (p = 0.603).

TABLE 4 - LOGIT MODEL OF SAH

Logit estimates

Number of obs =	8895
LR chi2(27) =	401.74
Prob > chi2 =	0.0000
Pseudo R2 =	0.0378

Log likelihood = -5115.757

yvar	Coef.	Std. Err.	z	P>|z|	[95% Conf.	Interval]
male	.0458014	.0582573	0.79	0.432	-.0683807	.1599835
age	-.0152439	.0039875	-3.82	0.000	-.0230592	-.0074286
age2	-.061195	.0143183	-4.27	0.000	-.0892584	-.0331316
age3	.2266146	.0477364	4.75	0.000	.133053	.3201761
ethbawi	-.5069956	.2188338	-2.32	0.021	-.935902	-.0780891
ethipb	-.4397762	.1944995	-2.26	0.024	-.8209882	-.0585642
ethothnw	-.6155907	.2739546	-2.25	0.025	-1.152532	-.0786495
part	.2914546	.0915696	3.18	0.001	.1119815	.4709278
unemp	-.2224889	.1086193	-2.05	0.041	-.4353788	-.0095989
retd	.0717155	.1051686	0.68	0.495	-.134411	.2778421
stdnt	.2235216	.2682633	0.83	0.405	-.3022649	.7493081
keephse	-.1366631	.0844388	-1.62	0.106	-.3021601	.028834
lsch14u	-.3551048	.141217	-2.51	0.012	-.631885	-.0783246
lsch14	-.3648383	.0896087	-4.07	0.000	-.5404682	-.1892084
lsch15	-.2420453	.0740448	-3.27	0.001	-.3871705	-.0969201
lsch17	.0929873	.1026102	0.91	0.365	-.1081249	.2940996
lsch18	.4843371	.1163431	4.16	0.000	.2563088	.7123653
lsch19	-.01383	.2273481	-0.06	0.951	-.4594241	.431764
regsc1s	.5064417	.1361412	3.72	0.000	.2396098	.7732735
regsc2	.4019567	.0724685	5.55	0.000	.259921	.5439925
regsc3n	.1699224	.0780869	2.18	0.030	.0168749	.3229699
regsc4	-.1159152	.0679944	-1.70	0.088	-.2491818	.0173515
regsc5n	-.3075666	.098354	-3.13	0.002	-.5003369	-.1147963
widow	-.2458365	.0932408	-2.64	0.008	-.4285852	-.0630878
single	-.1457644	.0835879	-1.74	0.081	-.3095937	.0180649
seprd	-.4221802	.1570441	-2.69	0.007	-.729981	-.1143794
divorce	-.3323718	.1225983	-2.71	0.007	-.57266	-.0920835
_cons	1.178291	.0903083	13.05	0.000	1.00129	1.355292

3.4 Results for the logit model

Tables 4 and 5 present the coefficient estimates and average and marginal effects for a logit model of self-assessed health (SAH). Here, the standard normal distribution of the probit model is replaced by a standard logistic function. Once again, the coefficients can only be given a qualitative interpretation and these qualitative effects follow the same pattern as the probit model. The marginal and average effects show the quantitative impact and can be compared directly with the linear probability and probit estimates. So, for example, the average effect of unemployment in the logit model is -0.046 (Table 5) compared with –0.047 for the probit model (Table 3) and –0.045 for the linear probability model (Table 1). The logit model also passes a RESET test with a chi-squared statistic of 0.08 (p=0.783).

TABLE 5 – AVERAGE AND MARGINAL EFFECTS FOR LOGIT MODEL

variable	dy/dx	X
male*	.0091059	.434401
age	-.0030348	.839460
age2	-.012183	3.13702
age3	.0451156	.242169
ethbawi*	-.1110924	.010455
ethipb*	-.0952794	.014390
ethothnw*	-.1371255	.007307
part*	.0550491	.121529
unemp*	-.0462216	.050590
retd*	.0141476	.221248
stdnt*	.042251	.011804
keephse*	-.0278002	.139966
lsch14u*	-.0756127	.036875
lsch15*	-.0493459	.271951
lsch17*	.018189	.088477
lsch18*	.087384	.088477
lsch19*	-.0027617	.013491
regsc1s*	.0901681	.056886
regsc2*	.0758616	.223834
regsc3n*	.0328796	.140866
regsc4*	-.0234723	.167285
regsc5n*	-.0647758	.060371
widow	-.0489424	.085779
single	-.0290195	.170770
seprd	-.0840498	.021585
divorce	-.0661703	.037549

(*) dy/dx is for discrete change of dummy variable from 0 to 1

. * RESET test;

chi2(1) =   0.08
        Prob > chi2 =   0.7826

4 The Ordered Probit Model

The empirical example in the previous section uses a binary measure of self-assessed health. This variable was created artificially by collapsing the underlying four-category scale where health could be assessed as either excellent, good, fair or poor. This is an example of a categorical variable where respondents are asked to report a particular category and where there is a natural ordering. It seems reasonable to assume that excellent health is better than good, which is better than fair, which is better than poor, for everyone in the population. An econometric model that can be used to deal with ordered categorical variables is the **ordered probit model**. This is designed to model a discrete dependent variable that takes ordered multinomial outcomes. For example, y = 0,1,2,3,..... It should be stressed that y is measured on an ordinal scale and the numerical values of y are arbitrary, except that they must be in ascending order.

The ordered probit model is an extension of the binary probit model (a similar extension is available for the logit model). Like the **binary probit** model, the ordered probit model can be expressed in terms of an underlying latent variable y*. Here this could be interpreted as the individual's 'true health'. The higher the value of y*, the more likely they are to report a higher category of self-assessed health. In our case there are four categories, so the range of values y* should be divided into four intervals, each one corresponding to a different category of self-assessed health. The *threshold values* (μ's) correspond to the cut-offs where an individual moves from reporting one category of self-assessed health to another. It is not possible to identify both the constant term and all of the cut-off points. So, in order to estimate the model, some of the threshold values (μ's) have to be fixed. The lowest value is set at minus infinity, the highest value is set at plus infinity and one other value has to be fixed. Conventionally, either the upper bound of the first interval (μ_1) is set equal to zero or the constant term is excluded from the regression model.

Like the binary probit model, explanatory variables are introduced into the model by making the latent variable y* a linear function of the X's, and adding a normally distributed error term. This means that the probability of an individual reporting a particular value of y = j is given by the difference between the probability of the respondent having a value of y* less than μ_j and the probability of having a value of y* less than μ_{j-1}. Using these probabilities it is possible to use maximum likelihood estimation to estimate the parameters of the model. These include the ß's (the coefficients on the X variables) and the unknown cut-off values (the μ's).

The ordered probit model applies when the threshold values (μ) are unknown. A variant on the model is **grouped data regression** or **interval regression**. This can be used when the values of thresholds are observed. For example, in many interview surveys individuals are presented with a range of categories and asked to state where their income lies. These categories are selected by the researcher and the upper and lower thresholds are known. Because the value of the μ's are known and do not have to be estimated, the estimates of the coefficients on the explanatory variables are more efficient. Also, because the values of the thresholds are in natural units, such as money, the predicted values from the grouped data regression are also measured in those units. This means that the grouped data regression is able to estimate the variance of the error term (σ^2) as well as the ß's. What is more, this scaling means that the latent variable is also measured in natural units and hence the coefficients measure marginal or average effects in natural units.

TABLE 6 - ORDERED PROBIT MODEL OF SAH

Ordered probit estimates

Log likelihood = -10163.906

	Number of obs	=	8895
	LR chi2(27)	=	399.67
	Prob > chi2	=	0.0000
	Pseudo R2	=	0.0193

yvar	Coef.	Std. Err.	z	P>|z|	[95% Conf.	Interval]
male	.0628071	.0281575	2.23	0.026	.0076195	.1179948
age	-.0060561	.0018943	-3.20	0.001	-.0097689	-.0023433
age2	-.028396	.0069248	-4.10	0.000	-.0419684	-.0148237
age3	.1069476	.0228589	4.68	0.000	.0621451	.1517502
ethbawi	-.1399885	.1138824	-1.23	0.219	-.3631939	.083217
ethipb	-.1968899	.0975955	-2.02	0.044	-.3881735	-.0056063
ethothnw	-.343557	.1358343	-2.53	0.011	-.6097873	-.0773267
part	.1887253	.0419252	4.50	0.000	.1065534	.2708972
unemp	-.1069106	.0551405	-1.94	0.053	-.2149841	.0011628
retd	.0416581	.0523803	0.80	0.426	-.0610054	.1443216
stdnt	.0248111	.1165797	0.21	0.831	-.2036809	.2533031
keephse	-.0802928	.0407453	-1.97	0.049	-.1601522	-.0004334
lsch14u	-.1815896	.0715292	-2.54	0.011	-.3217843	-.0413949
lsch14	-.1952184	.0430878	-4.53	0.000	-.279669	-.1107679
lsch15	-.0857022	.034904	-2.46	0.014	-.1541127	-.0172918
lsch17	.1004313	.0464239	2.16	0.031	.0094421	.1914204
lsch18	.145202	.0474957	3.06	0.002	.0521121	.2382918
lsch19	.0597935	.1039537	0.58	0.565	-.143952	.263539
regsc1s	.2095555	.057166	3.67	0.000	.0975122	.3215989
regsc2	.2018999	.0334748	6.03	0.000	.1362904	.2675094
regsc3n	.1167197	.0376377	3.10	0.002	.0429512	.1904881
regsc4	-.0599731	.0344098	-1.74	0.081	-.1274151	.0074688
regsc5n	-.1469187	.0510459	-2.88	0.004	-.2469668	-.0468706
widow	-.1094727	.0478125	-2.29	0.022	-.2031834	-.015762
single	-.0322312	.040252	-0.80	0.423	-.1111237	.0466613
seprd	-.1818617	.0798724	-2.28	0.023	-.3384087	-.0253147
divorce	-.1846496	.0614381	-3.01	0.003	-.305066	-.0642332
_cut1	-1.717435	.0471383		(Ancillary parameters)		
_cut2	-.6412847	.0436984				
_cut3	.7830036	.0438347				

RESET
(1) yf2 = 0.0

          chi2(1) =   5.20
       Prob > chi2 =   0.0226

Illustration of the ordered probit model

To illustrate the use of the ordered probit model, Table 6 shows estimates for the four-category measure of self-assessed health. The dependent variable is coded 0 for poor health, 1 for fair health, 2 for good health and 3 for excellent health. Table 6 includes the coefficients, their standard errors and z-ratios. It also includes estimates of the threshold parameters μ_1, μ_2 and μ_3 (labelled as _cut1, _cut2 and _cut3 in the table). These imply that a value of the latent variable less than −1.717 corresponds to poor health, a value between −1.717 and −0.641 corresponds to fair health, a value between −0.641 and 0.783 corresponds to good health and a value above 0.783 corresponds to excellent health. Notice that the predicted value of y* for the reference individual, where all of the explanatory variables equal zero, is zero. This value lies between −0.641 and 0.783, hence the reference individual would be predicted to report good health.

As for the binary probit model, the coefficients on the explanatory variables in the ordered probit model have a qualitative interpretation. A positive coefficient means that an individual has a higher value of latent health and is more likely to report a higher category of self-assessed health. A negative value means that they have a lower value of the latent variable and are likely to report a lower category of self-assessed health. As before, the results show a socio-economic gradient in self-assessed health. People in professional and managerial occupational groups have positive coefficients, while those in semi-skilled and unskilled occupations have negative coefficients. A similar gradient is apparent for levels of education. Because the threshold values are unknown, the latent variable and hence the coefficients are not measured in natural units. Like the binary probit model, quantitative predictions should be made on the basis of marginal effects for continuous explanatory variables and average effects for binary explanatory variables.

Once again, it is important to test the specification of the model before putting too much weight on the results. In fact a RESET test suggests that the model is mis-specified: the chi-squared is 5.20 ($p = 0.023$). This suggests that more work needs to be done to improve the specification of the model, perhaps by changing the way in which the explanatory variables are measured, by finding additional explanatory variables, or by splitting the sample into separate groups, perhaps by gender, or using a distribution other than the standard normal.

5 Multinomial Models

The **ordered probit model** discussed in the previous section applies to ordered categorical variables. Multinomial models apply to discrete dependent variables that can take unordered multinomial outcomes, for example, $y = 0,1,2,3,.....$. Again, the numerical values of y are arbitrary and in this case they do not imply any natural ordering of the outcomes. A classic example in economics is 'modal choice' in transport. There, the outcomes could represent different modes of transport, for example, bus, train, car, and the individual faces a choice of one of these mutually exclusive modes of transport for a particular journey. This choice will depend on the characteristics of the alternatives, such as price, convenience, quality of service and so on, and the characteristics of individuals, such as their levels of income. There is unlikely to be a natural ordering of the choices that applies to all individuals in all situations. In health economics, multinomial models are often applied to the choice of health insurance plan or of health care provider. They could also be used to model a choice of a particular treatment regime for an individual patient.

The most commonly applied model is the **multinomial logit model**, which is a natural extension of the binary logit model. In the multinomial logit model, the probability of individual i choosing outcome j, is given by:

$$P_{ij} = \exp(x_i\beta_j) / \Sigma_k \exp(x_i\beta_k) \tag{5}$$

Notice that the coefficients on the explanatory variables, β_j, are allowed to vary across the choices, j. So, for example, the impact of price could be different for different modes of transport, or the impact of co-payments could be different for different health insurance packages. It is not possible to identify separate ß's for all of the choices. To deal with this it is conventional to set the ß's for one of the outcomes equal to zero. This normalisation reflects the fact that only relative probabilities can be identified with respect to some base-line alternative. For example, in a model of hospital utilisation, where the possible outcomes are:

- no-use of hospital services;
- use of hospital outpatient services;
- use of hospital inpatient services;

no-use may be treated as the base-line category. The multinomial logit model would identify the probability of using outpatient services relative to no use and the probability of using inpatient services relative to no use.

The multinomial logit model is well-established and widely available in computer software packages. However, it is a restrictive specification and, in particular, it implies the *independence of irrelevant alternatives' (IIA)* property. To see this, consider the ratio of the probabilities of choosing two specific alternatives, j and l,

$$P_{ij}/P_{il} = [\exp(x_i\beta_j) / \Sigma_k \exp(x_i\beta_k)]/[\exp(x_i\beta_l) / \Sigma_k \exp(x_i\beta_k)] \qquad (6)$$
$$= \exp(x_i\beta_j)/\exp(x_i\beta_l)$$

This shows that the relative probability only depends on the characteristics of the two choices, j and l, and not on any of the other choices available. This implies that if a new alternative is introduced all of the absolute probabilities will be reduced proportionately. For example, consider the case of an individual choosing between a branded drug (brand X) and a generic alternative (generic A). Let us say that, faced with this choice, the probability of choosing brand X is 0.5 and the probability of choosing generic A is 0.5. The relative probability is therefore 0.5/0.5 = 1. Now we introduce a third option, a new generic B that shares the same characteristics as generic A. If the two generic drugs are perfect substitutes for each other, we might expect that the probability of choosing brand X will remain 0.5 and the probability of choosing the generics will be reduced to 0.25 each. But this contradicts the independence of irrelevant alternatives property, as the relative probability of choosing brand X compared to generic A will be increased to 0.5/0.25 = 2. In order to satisfy the IIA property, all of the absolute probabilities need to change so that all equal 0.333 and the relative probabilities remain constant. Many authors argue that the IIA property is too restrictive for many applications of multinomial models. The IIA property can be relaxed by using either a nested multinomial logit specification or a multinomial probit specification (see Jones, 2000, for further details).

It is possible to use the multinomial logit model to test whether the IIA property is appropriate. This test will work with three or more alternatives. The basic idea is to estimate the model with all of the alternatives and then to re-estimate it dropping one or more of the alternatives. The estimated coefficients should not change when an alternative is dropped and so a comparison of the two sets of results can be used to test for the property.

6 The Bivariate Probit Model

The ordered and multinomial models discussed in the previous two sections deal with dependent variables that can have different categorical outcomes. However, in both cases, there is a single underlying outcome variable. In contrast, the **bivariate probit model** provides a way of dealing with two separate binary dependent variables. Essentially it takes two independent binary probit models and estimates them together, allowing for a correlation between the error terms of the two equations. The practical application discussed here uses the HALS data to estimate the probability of someone reporting 'good' or 'excellent' self-assessed health together with the probability of them being a current smoker. Allowing for correlation between the error terms of the two equations recognises that there may be unobservable characteristics of individuals that influence both whether they smoke and their self-assessed health.

Given that the bivariate probit model is a natural extension of the binary probit model, it is possible to think about the bivariate model in terms of two latent variables, say, y^*_1 and y^*_2. Each of the latent variables is assumed to be a linear function of a set of explanatory variables, which may or may not be the same for the two equations, and each equation contains an error term. Like the binary probit model, these error terms are assumed to be normally distributed but they come from a joint or bivariate normal distribution. The bivariate distribution allows for a non-zero correlation between the errors. In other words, it is not assumed that the two error terms are independent of each other.

With two binary variables four possible outcomes can be observed. In the example here, these are a smoker who reports good or excellent health, a smoker who reports poor or fair health, a non-smoker who reports good or excellent health, or a non-smoker who reports fair or poor health. These correspond to different values of the latent variables y^*_1 and y^*_2 (remember that y^* is positive for a participant and non-positive for a non-participant). Using the assumption that the error terms are bivariate normal, it is possible to write down the probability of each of these four outcomes as a function of the explanatory variables and the unknown parameters of the model. This allows the model to be estimated by maximum likelihood methods. Because the outcomes are estimated jointly, it is possible not only to identify the slope coefficients for each of the two sets of explanatory variables but also the coefficient of correlation between the two error terms (ρ).

As with the binary probit model, the latent variables – and hence the ß's – are not measured in natural units and can only be given a qualitative interpretation but, like the binary probit model, marginal and average effects can be calculated. There is now a range of options for interpreting the results. Firstly, the same formulas as used for the binary probit marginal and average effects can be used for the bivariate probit. This gives the impact of a change of one of the explanatory variables on the *marginal* probability of each outcome, for example, the probability of someone being a smoker, or the probability of someone being in good or excellent health. Secondly, it is possible to calculate the marginal effect of an explanatory variable on the *joint* probability of each of the four outcome combinations, for example the probability that an individual is both a smoker and in good or excellent health. Finally, it is possible to calculate the marginal effects of the explanatory variables on *conditional* probabilities, for example the probability that someone reports good or excellent health, given that they are a smoker.

Table 7 shows the results for the bivariate probit model of smoking and self-assessed health estimated using the same set of explanatory variables as before. The coefficient estimates for both equations are broadly similar to those obtained using binary probit models. The equation for regular smoking shows that those in professional and managerial socio-economic groups are less likely to be smokers, while those in unskilled manual occupations are more likely to be smokers. Similarly, those who left school at 18 are less likely to be smokers, while those who left school before 16 are more likely to be smokers. The socio-economic gradient is once again apparent for self-assessed health with those in professional and managerial occupations more likely to report good or excellent health and those in unskilled and semi-skilled occupations less likely to report good or excellent health. The new information provided by the bivariate probit model is the estimate of ρ (rho), the correlation coefficient for the two error terms. The estimate is –0.172 and the chi-squared test statistic of 84.06 (p = 0.000) shows that this estimate is significantly different from zero. This is a plausible result that indicates that unobservable factors that are positively related to smoking are negatively related to good health.

TABLE 7 - BIVARIATE PROBIT MODEL OF SMOKING AND SAH

```
Bivariate probit regression                    Number of obs   =        8895
                                               Wald chi2(54)   =      961.06
Log likelihood = -10380.573                    Prob > chi2     =      0.0000
```

	Coef.	Std. Err.	z	P>|z|	[95% Conf.	Interval]
y1 (SAH)						
male	.0287978	.0348825	0.83	0.409	-.0395705	.0971662
age	-.0090962	.002365	-3.85	0.000	-.0137314	-.0044609
age2	-.0365567	.0085641	-4.27	0.000	-.0533421	-.0197714
age3	.1362723	.0284205	4.79	0.000	.0805691	.1919755
ethbawi	-.3057385	.1346342	-2.27	0.023	-.5696167	-.0418603
ethipb	-.2643758	.1175324	-2.25	0.024	-.494735	-.0340166
ethothnw	-.3633282	.1653823	-2.20	0.028	-.6874715	-.0391849
part	.1670081	.0535211	3.12	0.002	.0621088	.2719075
unemp	-.1389813	.066009	-2.11	0.035	-.2683565	-.009606
retd	.0366801	.0634862	0.58	0.563	-.0877505	.1611108
stdnt	.1194236	.1519335	0.79	0.432	-.1783606	.4172079
keephse	-.0774881	.0506601	-1.53	0.126	-.1767802	.021804
lsch14u	-.2147689	.0859358	-2.50	0.012	-.3832	-.0463379
lsch14	-.2191826	.053261	-4.12	0.000	-.3235723	-.114793
lsch15	-.1452899	.0437732	-3.32	0.001	-.2310839	-.059496
lsch17	.05568	.0597649	0.93	0.352	-.061457	.172817
lsch18	.2667823	.064975	4.11	0.000	.1394336	.3941309
lsch19	-.0177439	.1317902	-0.13	0.893	-.2760479	.2405602
regscls	.2906421	.0768606	3.78	0.000	.1399981	.441286
regsc2	.2364005	.0424117	5.57	0.000	.1532751	.3195259
regsc3n	.1023298	.0465678	2.20	0.028	.0110585	.1936011
regsc4	-.069094	.0414707	-1.67	0.096	-.1503751	.0121871
regsc5n	-.1918154	.0603343	-3.18	0.001	-.3100684	-.0735623
widow	-.15092	.0570616	-2.64	0.008	-.2627586	-.0390814
single	-.0861691	.0498545	-1.73	0.084	-.183882	.0115439
seprd	-.2501239	.0966591	-2.59	0.010	-.4395722	-.0606755
divorce	-.2027916	.074228	-2.73	0.006	-.3482757	-.0573074
_cons	.722309	.0536319	13.47	0.000	.6171923	.8274257

```
y2 (SMOKE)   |
      male |   .0553883    .0346972     1.60   0.110    -.0126169    .1233935
       age |  -.0081113    .0023966    -3.38   0.001    -.0128086   -.0034141
      age2 |    -.03637    .0085135    -4.27   0.000    -.0530562   -.0196838
      age3 |  -.0504658      .03064    -1.65   0.100    -.1105191    .0095876
   ethbawi |  -.3310786    .1431177    -2.31   0.021    -.6115841   -.0505731
    ethipb |  -.2997154    .1261894    -2.38   0.018    -.5470421   -.0523888
  ethothnw |   .1957156    .1649357     1.19   0.235    -.1275523    .5189835
      part |  -.0694085    .0509684    -1.36   0.173    -.1693047    .0304876
     unemp |   .3847182    .0650261     5.92   0.000     .2572693    .5121671
      retd |   .0583059     .065077     0.90   0.370    -.0692427    .1858545
     stdnt |  -.2108295    .1557235    -1.35   0.176     -.516042     .094383
   keephse |   .0046992    .0493621     0.10   0.924    -.0920488    .1014472
   lsch14u |   .2546079    .0907126     2.81   0.005     .0768143    .4324014
    lsch14 |   .2478051    .0540179     4.59   0.000      .141932    .3536782
    lsch15 |   .2215362    .0422187     5.25   0.000     .1387892    .3042833
    lsch17 |   .0089813     .057649     0.16   0.876    -.1040086    .1219713
    lsch18 |  -.2461978    .0614527    -4.01   0.000     -.366643   -.1257527
    lsch19 |  -.0484965    .1319448    -0.37   0.713    -.3071036    .2101106
   regsc1s |   -.507897    .0770645    -6.59   0.000    -.6589406   -.3568533
    regsc2 |  -.2822696    .0412017    -6.85   0.000    -.3630233   -.2015158
   regsc3n |  -.2360586    .0463523    -5.09   0.000    -.3269074   -.1452097
    regsc4 |   .0407858    .0411539     0.99   0.322    -.0398744     .121446
   regsc5n |   .1580333    .0607571     2.60   0.009     .0389515     .277115
     widow |   .0672059    .0612781     1.10   0.273    -.0528969    .1873087
    single |   .0568438    .0492002     1.16   0.248    -.0395869    .1532744
     seprd |    .397851     .095015     4.19   0.000     .2116251     .584077
    divorce |   .3727787    .0722291     5.16   0.000     .2312123    .5143452
     _cons |  -.4207566    .0521887    -8.06   0.000    -.5230446   -.3184686
-------------+----------------------------------------------------------------
    /athrho |  -.1736459    .0190506    -9.11   0.000    -.2109844   -.1363073
-------------+----------------------------------------------------------------
       rho |  -.1719214    .0184875                     -.2079086   -.1354694
-----------------------------------------------------------------------------
Likelihood ratio test of rho=0:     chi2(1) =   84.0588     Prob > chi2 = 0.0000
```

7 The Selection Problem

7.1 Identification

Sample selection bias arises when there are missing data for the dependent variable of interest. Recall the discussion of **item non-response** in the introduction. For example, in the HALS data set, measures of physiological health were collected at the nurse visit but not all of the original interviewees agreed to participate in the nurse visit. Models of health outcome (for example, forced expiratory volume (FEV)) could be estimated on the sample of individuals who responded to the nurse visit. But the selection problem means that it may not be possible to make inferences about the determinants of health outcome in the population as a whole. If there are systematic differences between the type of individuals who respond and those who do not, analysts are faced by a fundamental problem of identification.

For each individual in the HALS dataset, we know whether or not they responded to the nurse visit, and we know the characteristics of those who responded and those who did not. We also have a measure of the health outcome for those who responded and their associated characteristics. This means we could estimate the probability of responding conditional on the explanatory variables, and we can estimate the expected value of FEV, conditional upon the characteristics and on the fact that the individual agreed to participate. The identification problem arises because there is no way of knowing the FEV score that would have been reported by any individual who refused to participate in the nurse visit. They could have reported any logically feasible value of FEV. The fact that it is not possible to observe the outcomes of the non-responders means that in general it is not possible to identify the expected value of the outcome in the population as a whole. In other words, it is not possible to identify the population regression function, $E(y|X)$.

At a fundamental level this identification problem is insurmountable. However, inferences can be made if the analyst is willing to impose some assumptions on their model and data. Traditionally, the statistical literature often assumes independence or *ignorable non-response*. This is a strong assumption that asserts that those individuals who do not respond would behave in the same way as those who do respond, conditional upon the explanatory variables. Not only is this a strong assumption, it is not possible to test its validity. In the kind of observational health surveys often used in health economics it is unlikely to be tenable. For example, the reasons why an individual decides not to participate in the nurse visit may be correlated with unobservable factors that also influence their health outcome. This would violate the assumption of ignorable non-response and lead to potential selection bias. Participating in the nurse visit is time consuming and it may be that those who suspect they may benefit more from the visit, due to pre-existing chronic conditions, may be more willing to take part. Of course, this also means that their health outcomes are likely to be poorer than those who are not willing to participate.

The selection problem can be dealt with if the analyst is willing to impose identifying restrictions on their model. This involves making assumptions about the functional form of the regression model, excluding some explanatory variables that predict non-response from the equations that predict the outcome variable, and also assumptions about the distribution of the error terms in the two equations. In the econometrics literature the traditional approach to the selection problem has been a parametric approach, based on the so-called **Heckit** model, first introduced by James Heckman (see for example Heckman, 1979). This uses linear regression equations and assumes that the error terms have a normal distribution. However, recent years have seen the development of less restrictive **semiparametric** estimators which relax some, though not all, of the identifying restrictions (see Jones, 2000).

7.2 The Heckit model

The sample selection model consists of two equations. The first is a probit-type equation that predicts whether or not somebody responds. The second is a linear regression equation conditional on the individual providing a response. If it is assumed that the error terms of the two equations come from a bivariate normal distribution, which allows for a correlation between the two error terms and therefore the possibility of sample selection bias, the model can be estimated by maximum likelihood estimation.

In practice, the model is often estimated by a simpler two-step procedure. The first step is to estimate a probit equation for non-response and to save the residuals from this equation, these are known in the statistical literature as the **inverse Mill's ratio**. The inverse Mill's ratio is then added as an extra variable in the second stage regression of the outcome y on the set of explanatory variables. This second regression is estimated on the sub-sample of usable responses. Identification of the Heckit model can rely on finding some explanatory variables that enter the probit equation but do not enter the second stage regression. In the example given here, these are variables that influence whether somebody is willing to participate in the nurse visit, but do not influence their health outcome. In practice, it is often difficult to find such plausible identification restrictions, in which case the Heckit model is sometimes estimated with the same set of regressors in each equation. Then, identification relies on the non-linearity of the inverse Mill's ratio. It is worth mentioning that a test of whether the coefficient of the inverse Mill's ratio in the second stage regression is significantly different from zero, also provides a test for the existence of sample selection bias. This test is given by the t-ratio associated with the inverse Mill's ratio – a large value provides evidence of selection bias.

In practice, relying on identification by functional form is highly problematic. A plot of the inverse Mill's ratio shows that it is approximately linear for much of its range. The inverse Mills ratio is a function of the linear index (Xß) from the probit equation. This means that the range of the linear index, and hence of the explanatory variables in the probit equation, is important. It also means that the degree of censoring – in other words, the proportion of non-responders in the sample – is important, as this reduces the range of the observed values of the linear index. Leung and Yu (1996) reviewed the performance of the sample selection model and concluded that it depends on the collinearity between the inverse Mill's ratio and the explanatory variables in the regression equation. This arises if there are few or no regressors excluded from the second-stage regression, there is a high degree of non-response, there is low variability among the regressors in the probit equation or there is a large degree of unexplained variation in the probit equation. Leung and Yu recommend that applied researchers should always check for collinearity. A simple way of doing this is to regress the inverse Mills ratio on the explanatory variables from the outcome equation and examine the goodness of fit of this equation.

8 Count Data Regression

The measure of self-assessed health used in previous sections is an example of an ordered categorical variable. For convenience this was coded as y = 0, 1, 2, ... but these numerical values are arbitrary. *Count data regression* applies to dependent variables coded in the same way, where the values are meaningful in themselves, in other words, where the dependent variable represents a count of events. Common examples in health economics include measures of health care utilisation, such as the number of times an individual visits their doctor during a given period, or the number of prescriptions dispensed to an individual. Count data regression is appropriate when the dependent variable is a non-negative integer valued count, y = 0,1,2,..., where y is measured in natural units on a fixed scale. Typically, count data regression is applied when the distribution of the dependent variable is skewed. The data will usually contain a large proportion of zero observations, for example those who make no use of health care during the survey period, as well as a long right hand tail of individuals who make particularly heavy use of health care.

The basic statistical model for count data assumes that the probability of an event occurring (λ) during a brief period of time is constant and proportional to the duration of time. λ is known as the *intensity of the process*. The starting point for count data regression is the *Poisson process*. In order to turn this into an econometric model where the outcome y depends on a set of explanatory variables X, it is usually assumed that $\lambda = \exp(X\beta)$. The exponential function is used to ensure that the intensity of the process, which can also be interpreted as the mean number of events, given X, is always positive.

An important feature of the **Poisson regression** model is the *equi-dispersion property*. This means that the mean of y, given X, equals the variance of y, given X. For the Poisson model to be appropriate, this assumption should be reflected in the observed data. In practice, the distribution of many of the variables of interest to health economists, such as measures of health care utilisation, display *over-dispersion*. In other words, the mean of the variable is smaller than the variance of the variable. Many of the recent developments of count data regression have aimed to relax this restrictive feature of the Poisson model and to introduce models that allow for under- or over-dispersion in the data.

Two basic approaches are used to estimate count data regressions. Once the probability of a given count is specified, it is possible to use maximum likelihood estimation. This uses the fully specified probability distribution and maximises a sample likelihood function. The maximum likelihood approach builds in the assumption that the conditional mean of the dependent variable has the exponential form described above. It also builds in other features of the distribution such as the equi-dispersion property of the Poisson model. If the conditional mean specification is correct but there is under- or over-dispersion in the data, then maximum likelihood estimates of the standard errors of the regression coefficients and the t-tests will be biased. However, count data regressions have a convenient property that, as long as the conditional mean is correctly specified, maximum likelihood estimates of the ß's will be **consistent**. This is true even if other assumptions about the distribution, such as equi-dispersion are invalid.

The definition of the intensity of the process tells us that the mean of y, given X, is an exponential function of a linear index in the explanatory variables. This has the form of a non-linear regression function and means that count data models can also be estimated using a least squares approach. In particular, many recent applications of count data models use the **generalised method of moments (GMM)** estimator. This approach only rests on the assumption that the conditional mean is correctly specified, rather than the full probability distribution, and is therefore more robust than maximum likelihood estimation.

TABLE 8 - POISSON REGRESSION

Poisson regression

```
Number of obs   =       8881
LR chi2(27)     =   11237.48
Prob > chi2     =     0.0000
```

Log likelihood = -60409.332

```
Pseudo R2       =     0.0851
```

yvar	Coef.	Std. Err.	z	P>|z|	[95% Conf. Interval]	
male	.2084821	.0117404	17.76	0.000	.1854714	.2314928
age	-.0105308	.000819	-12.86	0.000	-.012136	-.0089255
age2	-.0839595	.0028981	-28.97	0.000	-.0896397	-.0782793
age3	-.0487911	.0117997	-4.13	0.000	-.0719181	-.0256641
ethbawi	-.8141589	.0616801	-13.20	0.000	-.9350497	-.6932681
ethipb	-.5500904	.049943	-11.01	0.000	-.6479769	-.4522039
ethothnw	-.0063454	.0584604	-0.11	0.914	-.1209257	.1082348
part	-.1064703	.0170825	-6.23	0.000	-.1399513	-.0729893
unemp	.2894559	.017382	16.65	0.000	.2553877	.323524
retd	-.0306639	.0231153	-1.33	0.185	-.0759691	.0146413
stdnt	-.3541118	.0680278	-5.21	0.000	-.4874439	-.2207797
keephse	-.0282476	.0161667	-1.75	0.081	-.0599337	.0034384
lsch14u	.4431014	.0303888	14.58	0.000	.3835405	.5026623
lsch14	.332869	.0182712	18.22	0.000	.297058	.3686799
lsch15	.2827287	.0134964	20.95	0.000	.2562763	.3091812
lsch17	-.0124955	.0204422	-0.61	0.541	-.0525614	.0275704
lsch18	-.4090868	.0239678	-17.07	0.000	-.4560629	-.3621107
lsch19	-.280291	.0527058	-5.32	0.000	-.3835926	-.1769895
regsc1s	-.6155476	.0305427	-20.15	0.000	-.6754102	-.555685
regsc2	-.2591576	.0139296	-18.60	0.000	-.2864591	-.231856
regsc3n	-.2963375	.0161676	-18.33	0.000	-.3280254	-.2646496
regsc4	.0402827	.012723	3.17	0.002	.015346	.0652194
regsc5n	.1951064	.0175924	11.09	0.000	.160626	.2295869
widow	.1033594	.0225812	4.58	0.000	.059101	.1476178
single	.0455864	.015946	2.86	0.004	.0143329	.0768399
seprd	.5266067	.024033	21.91	0.000	.4795029	.5737105
divorce	.3720886	.0195796	19.00	0.000	.3337133	.410464
_cons	1.698063	.0173809	97.70	0.000	1.663997	1.732129

Example of a Poisson regression

Table 8 shows an example of the **Poisson regression model**. The dependent variable is the number of cigarettes smoked per day by respondents to the HALS. Respondents are asked to report the actual number of cigarettes and the variable can be interpreted as a count. The model estimates the number of cigarettes smoked as a function of the usual list of explanatory variables. Table 8 reports the coefficients, standard errors and implied z-ratios for each of the variables. Recall that the coefficients relate to the intensity of the process, which is a non-linear function of the X's. So the ß's are not measured in the original units of the count data and inferences about the impact of a particular variable on the actual number of counts have to be made by re-transforming the coefficient estimates. However, we can use the coefficients to analyse the qualitative impacts of the variables. So, for example, the results show a strong socio-economic gradient in the number of cigarettes smoked, with those in professional and managerial occupations having negative coefficients and the variables for semi-skilled and unskilled occupations having positive coefficients.

Inferences about quantitative effects can be made by calculating the marginal effect for a continuous explanatory variable, say X_k, which is given by the formula:

$$\partial E(y|X)/\partial X_k = \beta_k \exp(X\beta) \tag{7}$$

while the formula for the average effect of a binary variable is:

$$E(y| X_k =1) - E(y| X_k =0) = \exp(X\beta| X_k =1) - \exp(X\beta| X_k =0) \tag{8}$$

As with binary choice models, it is clear that these marginal and average effects depend on the values of the other explanatory variables. Again, standard practice is to evaluate these at the mean of the other X's but estimates can be calculated for every individual in the sample. Average and marginal effects are given in Table 9.

TABLE 9 – AVERAGE AND MARGINAL EFFECTS FOR POISSON REGRESSION

```
Marginal effects after poisson
     y = predicted number of events (predict)
       =  4.6479522
```

variable	dy/dx	X
male*	.984229	.433960
age	-.0489466	.841797
age2	-.3902397	3.13685
age3	-.2267785	.241804
ethbawi*	-2.611021	.010472
ethipb*	-1.982213	.014413
ethothnw*	-.0294013	.007319
part*	-.4755526	.121608
unemp*	1.537752	.050332
retd*	-.1413172	.221371
stdnt*	-1.391851	.011823
keephse*	-.1299703	.140187
lsch14u*	2.549311	.036933
lsch15*	1.406401	.271704
lsch17*	-.0577811	.088616
lsch18*	-1.618129	.088616
lsch19*	-1.140367	.013287
regscls*	-2.212712	.056976
regsc2*	-1.124598	.224186
regsc3n*	-1.242925	.141088
regsc4*	.1897727	.167098
regsc5n*	.989656	.060241
widow	.4804094	.085801
single	.2118833	.170701
seprd	2.447643	.021619
divorce	1.72945	.037496

(*) dy/dx is for discrete change of dummy variable from 0 to 1

TABLE 10 - NEGATIVE BINOMIAL MODEL

```
Negative binomial regression                          Number of obs    =       8881
                                                      LR chi2(27)      =     263.52
                                                      Prob > chi2      =     0.0000
Log likelihood = -17697.843                           Pseudo R2        =     0.0074
```

yvar	Coef.	Std. Err.	z	P>|z|	[95% Conf.	Interval]
male	.239186	.0758291	3.15	0.002	.0905638	.3878083
age	-.0085022	.0050999	-1.67	0.095	-.0184979	.0014935
age2	-.0813607	.0186917	-4.35	0.000	-.1179958	-.0447256
age3	-.0419942	.0614688	-0.68	0.494	-.1624708	.0784824
ethbawi	-.7740075	.3144606	-2.46	0.014	-1.390339	-.157676
ethipb	-.6184399	.2669483	-2.32	0.021	-1.141649	-.0952308
ethothnw	-.0107198	.3696925	-0.03	0.977	-.7353038	.7138643
part	-.1351946	.1108069	-1.22	0.222	-.3523721	.0819829
unemp	.2971866	.1482682	2.00	0.045	.0065862	.587787
retd	-.054419	.1367701	-0.40	0.691	-.3224835	.2136454
stdnt	-.4090891	.3164427	-1.29	0.196	-1.029305	.2111273
keephse	-.0458872	.1086378	-0.42	0.673	-.2588134	.167039
lsch14u	.3767383	.1958954	1.92	0.054	-.0072097	.7606862
lsch14	.2157437	.1177754	1.83	0.067	-.0150919	.4465793
lsch15	.2576711	.0947917	2.72	0.007	.0718827	.4434594
lsch17	.0042482	.125851	0.03	0.973	-.2424153	.2509116
lsch18	-.393168	.1300719	-3.02	0.003	-.6481042	-.1382317
lsch19	-.3720131	.2830083	-1.31	0.189	-.9266991	.1826729
regsc1s	-.5046795	.1601508	-3.15	0.002	-.8185692	-.1907897
regsc2	-.2879881	.0893091	-3.22	0.001	-.4630307	-.1129455
regsc3n	-.3526389	.1020198	-3.46	0.001	-.5525941	-.1526838
regsc4	-.0033635	.0924934	-0.04	0.971	-.1846472	.1779203
regsc5n	.1644896	.1372828	1.20	0.231	-.1045797	.4335589
widow	.1867993	.1330337	1.40	0.160	-.0739419	.4475405
single	.0685149	.1077326	0.64	0.525	-.142637	.2796669
seprd	.5293877	.2140531	2.47	0.013	.1098514	.9489241
divorce	.4541375	.164771	2.76	0.006	.1311923	.7770826
_cons	1.729985	.1163724	14.87	0.000	1.501899	1.958071
/lnalpha	2.111045	.0227965			2.066364	2.155725
alpha	8.256861	.1882273			7.896063	8.634146

```
Likelihood ratio test of alpha=0:  chibar2(01) = 8.5e+04 Prob>=chibar2 = 0.000
```

Over-dispersion and 'excess zeros'

The results in Table 8 are estimated by maximum likelihood, assuming that the Poisson distribution is appropriate for the data on the number of cigarettes smoked. In fact, this is unlikely to be valid. In particular, there is a very high proportion of zeros in the observed data. Around 70% of individuals were not current smokers at the time of the HALS survey. Among other things, this means that the conditional mean of the data does not equal the conditional variance and leads us to look for specifications that allow for **over-dispersion** and what are known as **'excess zeros'**. In other words, the data exhibit a higher frequency of zero observations than would be predicted by the simple Poisson model.

One possible explanation for over-dispersion and excess zeros is additional individual heterogeneity beyond differences that can be summarised by the observed explanatory variables. Mullahy (1997) emphasises that the presence of excess zeros in count data can be seen as a strict implication of unobservable heterogeneity. Up to now individual differences only enter the model through differences in the X variables. If there are additional unobservable differences across individuals, these could be added as an extra unobservable variable or error term. The effect of adding this further heterogeneity is to spread out the distribution of the count variable, meaning that more observations are shifted to the tails of the distribution so that we would expect to observe more zero values and more high values than would be predicted by the simple Poisson model.

The most commonly applied model that allows for additional unobservable heterogeneity is the negative binomial or **negbin model**. This allows for over-dispersion by assuming that the individual error term comes from a particular probability distribution (the **gamma distribution**). By doing this, it is possible to write down a new probability function for y and hence to estimate the model by maximum likelihood estimation. This new model is more flexible and relaxes the equi-dispersion property of the Poisson model. Two special cases of the negbin model are typically estimated in practice: one in which the variance of y is proportional to the mean of y and the other in which the variance is a quadratic function of the mean. An attractive feature of the negbin model is that it nests the Poisson model as a special case and this can be tested using a conventional t-test on the coefficient that reflects over-dispersion. The negative binomial model has been applied extensively in studies of health care utilisation (see Jones, 2000, for a review of this literature).

TABLE 11 - ZERO INFLATED NEGBIN MODEL I

```
Zero-inflated negative binomial regression        Number of obs   =      8881
                                                  Nonzero obs     =      2914
                                                  Zero obs        =      5967

Inflation model = logit                           LR chi2(27)     =    291.89
Log likelihood  = -15749.16                       Prob > chi2     =    0.0000
```

yvar	Coef.	Std. Err.	z	P>|z|	[95% Conf.	Interval]
yvar						
male	.165783	.024712	6.71	0.000	.1173485	.2142176
age	-.002588	.001747	-1.48	0.138	-.006012	.000836
age2	-.0421808	.006039	-6.98	0.000	-.0540171	-.0303445
age3	.0558082	.0240881	2.32	0.021	.0085965	.1030199
ethbawi	-.4568471	.1134162	-4.03	0.000	-.6791388	-.2345553
ethipb	-.2997162	.0999778	-3.00	0.003	-.4956691	-.1037632
ethothnw	-.228455	.1164398	-1.96	0.050	-.4566728	-.0002371
part	-.0354273	.0357876	-0.99	0.322	-.1055697	.0347152
unemp	-.0225922	.037748	-0.60	0.550	-.096577	.0513926
retd	-.1184293	.0466222	-2.54	0.011	-.2098071	-.0270515
stdnt	-.1078132	.1348282	-0.80	0.424	-.3720717	.1564453
keephse	-.0310741	.0338928	-0.92	0.359	-.0975028	.0353547
lsch14u	.1087141	.065943	1.65	0.099	-.0205318	.2379601
lsch14	.0246182	.0393796	0.63	0.532	-.0525645	.1018009
lsch15	.0458843	.0293772	1.56	0.118	-.011694	.1034626
lsch17	-.0176921	.0432019	-0.41	0.682	-.1023662	.066982
lsch18	-.0963355	.0500321	-1.93	0.054	-.1943966	.0017257
lsch19	-.2110032	.1064913	-1.98	0.048	-.4197223	-.0022841
regsc1s	.0646949	.0667196	0.97	0.332	-.066073	.1954628
regsc2	.033021	.0300546	1.10	0.272	-.0258849	.0919268
regsc3n	-.0642388	.0339188	-1.89	0.058	-.1307185	.0022409
regsc4	-.0116592	.0271075	-0.43	0.667	-.064789	.0414706
regsc5n	.0404697	.0379354	1.07	0.286	-.0338823	.1148218
widow	.0449928	.0464207	0.97	0.332	-.04599	.1359757
single	.0033871	.0336483	0.10	0.920	-.0625624	.0693366
seprd	.1752159	.0547423	3.20	0.001	.067923	.2825088
divorce	.0554193	.0429662	1.29	0.197	-.0287929	.1396315
_cons	2.808045	.0372049	75.48	0.000	2.735124	2.880965
inflate						
_cons	.7144212	.0226187	31.59	0.000	.6700895	.758753
/lnalpha	-1.527933	.035427	-43.13	0.000	-1.597369	-1.458498
alpha	.2169836	.0076871			.2024284	.2325854

Table 10 shows estimates of a negbin model for the number of cigarettes smoked. The conditional mean function for the negbin model is still an exponential function of the explanatory variables and the coefficients should be interpreted in just the same way as the Poisson model. The additional parameter, α (alpha), estimates the degree of over-dispersion in the data. This parameter is large (8.257) and highly significant (with p = 0.000). In this example there is strong evidence to reject the Poisson specification as a special case of the negbin. The qualitative results for the negbin model are broadly comparable with those of the Poisson model, so that, for example, we again see a socio-economic gradient in the level of smoking. But there are some small changes in the magnitudes of the coefficients and substantial changes in the standard errors and z-ratios.

Recall that our dependent variable is heavily influenced by a large proportion of zero observations – around 70% of the sample. It is likely that much of the distinction between smokers and non-smokers is now being picked up by the estimate of over-dispersion. However, like the Poisson model, the negbin model assumes that there is a single process underlying all of the observed values of the dependent variable, whether y equals 0 or is greater than 0. Other recent developments of count data regression have been based on the idea that there is something special about the zero observations and that they are not just a reflection of over-dispersion. This makes a qualitative distinction between participants and non-participants; for example, between those who use health care and those who do not, or between smokers and non-smokers. One example of this kind of approach are so-called *zero-inflated models*. These are an example of *mixture models*. They take a standard count-data model such as the Poisson or negative binomial and add extra weight to the probability of observing a zero value. This probability can be interpreted as a splitting mechanism that divides individuals into non-users, with a probability q, and potential users with probability 1-q. The probability q may be a function of a set of explanatory variables. So, in the zero-inflated model the probability of observing zero is made up of the probability of someone being a non-user plus the probability that they are a potential user, multiplied by the probability of observing a zero under the standard count data model.

Tables 11 and 12 show estimates of the *zero-inflated negative binomial regression* for the number of cigarettes smoked. The first set of results assumes the splitting mechanism is just a constant. The second allows explanatory variables to influence the splitting mechanism. These show evidence of a split between non-smokers and potential smokers

TABLE 12 - ZERO INFLATED NEGBIN MODEL II

```
. zinb yvar $xvars if wave==1, inflate($xvars _cons);
```

Zero-inflated negative binomial regression		
	Number of obs	=	8881
	Nonzero obs	=	2914
	Zero obs	=	5967

Inflation model = logit		LR chi2(27)	=	290.19
Log likelihood = -15419.93		Prob > chi2	=	0.0000

yvar	Coef.	Std. Err.	z	P>|z|	[95% Conf. Interval]
yvar						
male	.1651176	.0246702	6.69	0.000	.1167649	.2134702
age	-.0026078	.0017422	-1.50	0.134	-.0060225	.0008069
age2	-.0419216	.0060272	-6.96	0.000	-.0537346	-.0301085
age3	.0575564	.0238905	2.41	0.016	.0107319	.1043809
ethbawi	-.45416	.1130194	-4.02	0.000	-.6756739	-.2326462
ethipb	-.2975508	.09964	-2.99	0.003	-.4928415	-.1022601
ethothnw	-.2293836	.1163446	-1.97	0.049	-.4574148	-.0013524
part	-.0356723	.0357427	-1.00	0.318	-.1057266	.0343821
unemp	-.0229508	.0377367	-0.61	0.543	-.0969134	.0510119
retd	-.1196494	.0465099	-2.57	0.010	-.2108071	-.0284918
stdnt	-.1044109	.1341013	-0.78	0.436	-.3672447	.1584229
keephse	-.0312997	.033858	-0.92	0.355	-.0976602	.0350608
lsch14u	.1071627	.0657906	1.63	0.103	-.0217845	.2361099
lsch14	.0241309	.0393051	0.61	0.539	-.0529058	.1011675
lsch15	.0456296	.0293469	1.55	0.120	-.0118893	.1031485
lsch17	-.0178212	.0431329	-0.41	0.679	-.1023601	.0667177
lsch18	-.0951733	.0498875	-1.91	0.056	-.192951	.0026044
lsch19	-.209386	.106156	-1.97	0.049	-.4174478	-.0013241
regsc1s	.0660621	.0664783	0.99	0.320	-.064233	.1963573
regsc2	.0334974	.0300076	1.12	0.264	-.0253164	.0923112
regsc3n	-.0634174	.0338604	-1.87	0.061	-.1297825	.0029477
regsc4	-.0115948	.0270846	-0.43	0.669	-.0646796	.04149
regsc5n	.0403628	.0379119	1.06	0.287	-.0339431	.1146687
widow	.0443472	.0462971	0.96	0.338	-.0463935	.1350879
single	.0035342	.0336015	0.11	0.916	-.0623235	.0693919
seprd	.1748827	.0547107	3.20	0.001	.0676517	.2821136
divorce	.0549495	.042945	1.28	0.201	-.0292211	.1391201
_cons	2.808213	.0371605	75.57	0.000	2.735379	2.881046

```
inflate      |
      male   |  -.0942922    .0580971    -1.62   0.105    -.2081603     .019576
       age   |   .0127342    .0040913     3.11   0.002     .0047154    .0207531
      age2   |   .0620747    .0142394     4.36   0.000      .034166    .0899834
      age3   |   .1243065    .0547056     2.27   0.023     .0170856    .2315275
   ethbawi   |   .5341702    .2412783     2.21   0.027     .0612734    1.007067
    ethipb   |   .5119719    .2181043     2.35   0.019     .0844953    .9394484
  ethothnw   |  -.3434212    .2744485    -1.25   0.211    -.8813304     .194488
      part   |   .1044786    .0846668     1.23   0.217    -.0614652    .2704224
     unemp   |  -.6145025    .1056705    -5.82   0.000    -.8216129    -.407392
      retd   |  -.1293913    .1099201    -1.18   0.239    -.3448308    .0860481
     stdnt   |   .3740523    .2761051     1.35   0.175    -.1671037    .9152083
    keephse  |  -.0189792    .0813432    -0.23   0.816     -.178409    .1404506
    lsch14u  |  -.4630782    .1533632    -3.02   0.003    -.7636645   -.1624919
     lsch14  |  -.4331438    .0911224    -4.75   0.000    -.6117405   -.2545472
     lsch15  |  -.3681723    .0696687    -5.28   0.000    -.5047204   -.2316243
     lsch17  |  -.0140726     .096944    -0.15   0.885    -.2040793    .1759341
     lsch18  |    .429907    .1066641     4.03   0.000     .2208492    .6389647
     lsch19  |   .1317406    .2291932     0.57   0.565    -.3174699    .5809511
    regsc1s  |    .869616    .1368796     6.35   0.000     .6013368    1.137895
     regsc2  |   .4539897    .0690051     6.58   0.000     .3187422    .5892372
    regsc3n  |   .3767895    .0772583     4.88   0.000     .2253661    .5282129
     regsc4  |  -.0716924    .0671394    -1.07   0.286    -.2032833    .0598985
    regsc5n  |  -.2585987     .099083    -2.61   0.009    -.4527977   -.0643997
     widow   |  -.1072686    .1042935    -1.03   0.304    -.3116801    .0971429
    single   |  -.0822875    .0817644    -1.01   0.314    -.2425427    .0779677
     seprd   |  -.6518891    .1533489    -4.25   0.000    -.9524475   -.3513308
    divorce  |  -.6073318     .117501    -5.17   0.000    -.8376295   -.3770341
      _cons  |    .697431    .0869027     8.03   0.000     .5271048    .8677571
-------------+----------------------------------------------------------------
   /lnalpha  |  -1.530275    .0353395   -43.30   0.000    -1.599539   -1.461011
-------------+----------------------------------------------------------------
     alpha   |   .2164762    .0076502                      .2019897    .2320017
------------------------------------------------------------------------------
```

– the constant labelled *inflate* in Table 11 is statistically significant – and also that this split is influenced by observable explanatory variables – many of the variables that appear in the splitting equation, labelled *inflate* in Table 12, are statistically significant. Notice also that there are now substantial differences in both the sign and the size of the regression coefficients for the negbin regression model compared to the specification that did not allow for zero inflation (Table 10). For example, the negbin results in Tables 11 and 12 no longer show such a clear socio-economic gradient in the level of smoking. This suggests that the earlier results were largely driven by the distinction between smokers and non-smokers, and that effectively the count data regressions were acting like binary choice models, explaining whether someone smokes rather than how much they smoke.

The zero-inflated specification separates out the binary choice of whether to smoke or not from the number of cigarettes smoked given that someone is a smoker. Another way of dealing with this distinction between participants and non-participants is to use a so-called *hurdle* or *two-part specification*. This assumes that the participation decision and the positive values of the count data are generated by two separate probability functions. In some applications, the participation decision is modelled using a standard binary choice model such as the **logit** or **probit**. In others, a count data specification such as the **Poisson** or **negbin** model is used, with a dependent variable that can take values of either 0 or 1. Then a standard count data regression is applied to the sub-sample of participants, allowing for the fact that the count data are truncated at zero.

When faced with count data that exhibit over-dispersion and a large proportion of zero observations, analysts are faced with a choice of two types of specification: those that emphasise the role of unobservable heterogeneity, such as the negbin model; and those that emphasise the special role of zero observations, such as zero-inflated or hurdle models. Applications of zero-inflated or hurdle models often make the probability of participation a function of explanatory variables, as interest lies in the type of factors that distinguish users and non-users of health care, or smokers and non-smokers. Applications of the negbin model often treat over-dispersion as a fixed parameter and do not allow it to be a function of the explanatory variables. This may bias the comparison in favour of zero-inflated and hurdle models. The negbin model also relies on a specific functional form for the unobservable heterogeneity.

Recent work in the health economics literature has advocated a more robust and flexible approach, which treats unobservable heterogeneity in a non-parametric way. For example, Deb and Trivedi (1997) adopt a *finite mixture approach* to model health care utilisation (see the Technical Appendix for details). In this approach, the unobservable heterogeneity is treated as a discrete random variable, modelled by a series of dummy variables, where each category of the variable represents an unobservable 'type' of individual. So, for example, with a two-point mixture there would be two types, such as 'healthy' and 'ill' individuals.

In the finite mixture approach, the probability of an individual belonging to one of these types is estimated along with the other parameters of the model. Deb and Trivedi apply finite mixture models with two and three points of support for data on the demand for medical care among individuals aged 66 and over in the 1987 US medical care expenditure survey. Demand is measured by six different indicators of annual health care utilisation and the finite mixture model is compared to hurdle and zero-inflated specifications. The negbin models with two points of support are preferred on the basis of various statistical criteria. Deb and Trivedi interpret the points of support as two latent populations of 'healthy' and 'ill' individuals reflecting unobservable differences in frailty across the population.

9 Duration Analysis

The previous section discussed count data models, where the dependent variable is the number of events occurring over a period of time, for example the number of visits to a doctor during the previous month. A closely related topic is duration analysis. Here, the focus is on the time elapsed before an event occurs, rather than on the number of events. So, for example, duration could measure the number of years that someone lives from birth; or it could measure a patient's length of stay after admission to hospital; or it could measure the number of years that someone smoked cigarettes.

The HALS can be used to illustrate the application of duration analysis. Forster and Jones (2001) used duration analysis to explore two aspects of smoking: the decisions to start and to quit. Here, there are two measures of duration: the age at which somebody starts smoking cigarettes and the number of years that they smoke once they have started. By analysing these two variables we can learn about the impact of individual characteristics on the probability of starting and the probability of quitting smoking. Recall that the original HALS data were collected in 1984-85. The survey included information that allows individuals to be divided into those who were regular smokers at the time of the survey, those who had been regular smokers but had quit by the time of the survey and those who had never smoked prior to the survey.

The current and ex-smokers in the survey were asked how old they were when they started to smoke cigarettes. This is self-reported retrospective data and so may be prone to problems of measurement error, such as recall bias. Recall bias occurs when respondents have difficulty recalling events from their past, it includes phenomena such as 'telescoping' of events and 'heaping' of observations at round numbers.

For those who had started smoking at some time prior to the survey, we observe the actual value of duration and their age when they started smoking. For those individuals who had not smoked prior to the survey, there is a problem of *censoring*. In other words, all we know is that they had not started smoking prior to the date of the interview. It is possible that some of these individuals will go on to start smoking at a later age. All we know is that their age of starting is at least as great as their age at the time of the survey. For this reason we refer to them as *right censored* observations. So for these individuals we can use the probability that their true duration is greater than the censored value – in this case, their age at the time of the HALS. Standard models of duration data are built on the assumption that eventually everyone will 'fail'. In this application, this would mean that eventually all individuals will start smoking. This is unlikely to be plausible in the case of smoking and, as we shall see below, it is possible to relax the specification to allow some individuals to remain non-smokers.

For those who become smokers the second measure of duration is the number of years that they smoke. This helps us to analyse the probability of quitting. This new variable can be defined by taking the individuals' ages at the time of the interview and subtracting the ages that they started smoking. For those individuals who had already quit smoking prior to the survey, the number of years since they quit should also be subtracted. Once again, there is a problem of right censoring. For those individuals who had quit prior to the survey, we observe a complete spell. For those individuals who were still current smokers at the time of the survey, all we know is the age that they started and the fact that they are still smoking in 1984-85. For these individuals we can only estimate the probability that they have remained as smokers for at least that many years, given their characteristics.

The HALS data provide us with a third measure of duration. The survey respondents were linked with the NHS Central Register of Deaths, which provides information on survival rates. For respondents who had died by 1997, the survey provides information on their age and cause of death taken from death certificates. This third measure of duration is an individual's lifespan in years, with the origin defined as an individual's birth and the duration measured up to their age at death. Once again, there is a problem of right censoring. For those individuals who died between the collection of the HALS data in 1984 and the collection of the deaths data in 1997, we observe a complete spell. The majority of the original HALS respondents were still alive in 1997, and these represent right censored observations. But the deaths data raise a further issue, the problem of *left truncation*. The natural origin for the measure of lifespan is an individual's birth. However, the HALS was designed as a representative random sample of the living population in 1984. To be included in the survey, an individual must have survived at least to their age at the time of HALS. Individuals who were born and died prior to HALS are a form of missing data. For each age group the probability of surviving to the time of the survey may vary systematically across different types of individuals. This creates a source of bias – the problem of left truncation. To deal with this, the duration models need to be adapted to incorporate the probability that an individual survives at least to their age at the time of HALS.

Analysis of models of survival or duration revolves around the notion of a hazard function h(t). This measures the probability that someone fails at time t, given that they have survived up to that point. It can be written as:

$$h(t) = f(t)/S(t) \tag{9}$$

where the two components on the right-hand side are the probability density function (f(t)), the probability of failing at time t, and the survival function (S(t)), which is the probability that someone survives to at least time t. In estimating duration models, the density function is used for uncensored observations, where we observe their actual time of failure, and the survival function is used for censored observations where we only know they have survived at least to time t.

Parametric models of duration assume particular functional forms for f(t) and S(t) and therefore for the hazard function h(t). A common example is the **Weibull model**. The hazard function for the Weibull model takes the form,

$$h(t) = hpt^{p-1}. \exp(X\beta) \tag{10}$$

where h and p are parameters to be estimated. This develops the kind of regression model we have seen in previous sections in that it is not just a function of the explanatory variables X but also of duration itself (t). Duration analysis allows us to estimate the impact of individual characteristics (the X's) on the probability of failure. It also allows us to estimate how the hazard function changes with time. In the Weibull model the parameter p is known as the shape parameter. The hazard function is increasing for p > 1, showing *increasing duration dependence*, while it is decreasing for p < 1, showing *decreasing duration dependence*. Duration dependence may be of interest in itself. For example, we may want to learn whether the probability of someone receiving a job offer increases or decreases the longer they have been unemployed.

Parametric models rely on fully specifying the baseline hazard function. This assumption may not be valid and it is particularly vulnerable to problems caused by unobservable heterogeneity across individuals. A more flexible approach is to use a semiparametric model. The best known example is the **Cox proportional hazard**

model. This leaves the baseline hazard unspecified, treated as an unknown function of time. Because the method does not require specification of the baseline hazard, it is more robust than parametric approaches. In order to implement the method, the duration data are converted into a rank ordering of individuals according to their level of duration, t. Because this throws away information on the actual value of t, the method is less efficient than a parametric approach.

Analysis of the age of starting smoking is more complicated. As mentioned earlier, standard duration models assume that eventually everyone fails – in this case eventually everyone would start smoking. This seems to be an implausible assumption, and models based on the assumption do not do a good job of fitting the observed data. An alternative is to use a *split population model*. This augments the standard duration analysis by adding a splitting mechanism analogous to the zero-inflated models of count data. So, for example, a probit specification could be added to model the probability that somebody will eventually smoke. When this splitting mechanism is added to the duration model, it does a far better job of explaining the observed data on age of starting than models that omit a splitting mechanism (see Forster and Jones, 2001).

As with count data, dealing with unobservable heterogeneity is a particular preoccupation in the literature on duration models. The existence of *unobservable heterogeneity* will bias estimates of duration dependence. Unobservable heterogeneity can be dealt with by adding an extra error term to the model. Like count data models, this can be dealt with parametrically by assuming a particular functional form for the distribution of the error term. Alternatively, a non-parametric approach can be adopted, using the finite mixture model (see Section 8). This assumes that the unobservable error term has a discrete distribution characterised by a set of mass points, where the value of these mass points and the probabilities attached to them are estimated as part of maximum likelihood estimation (see for example Heckman and Singer, 1984).

10 Panel Data Models

10.1 Linear models

All of the models described so far have been applied to a single cross-section survey, where each individual is observed only once. With **panel data** a longitudinal element is added to the data and there are repeated measurements for each individual observation. Recall that the original HALS cross-section study was repeated seven years later in 1991-92. Rather than drawing a new random sample of individuals, the original HALS respondents were revisited and asked to complete the same face-to-face interview, nurse visit and postal questionnaire as in the original study. So, for each variable in the survey, and for each individual respondent, we observe two values. With only two waves, HALS is an example of a so-called 'short' panel where the number of individuals, n, is far greater than the number of waves, T. Longitudinal data add a new dimension to the analysis and allow researchers to explore the dynamics of individual behaviour. They also provide more scope for dealing with individual heterogeneity.

Consider a standard linear regression model in which there are repeated measurements (t = 1,....,T) for a sample of n individuals (i = 1,....,n),

$$y_{it} = X_{it}\beta + \mu_i + \epsilon_{it} \tag{11}$$

Here the dependent variable y is observed for individual, i, in each of the waves, t. Similarly, the explanatory variables X are observed at each wave. Some of these variables will be time varying (for example, an individual's income at different points of time). Others may be fixed or time invariant (such as an individual's gender or ethnic background). The error term of the regression equation (11) has been split into two components (this is known as an **error components model**). The first term, μ_i, is an individual-specific unobservable effect – the characteristics of the individual i that remain constant over time. The second term, ϵ_{it}, is a random error term representing idiosyncratic shocks that vary over time. Typically, it is assumed that μ_i and ϵ_{it} are uncorrelated with each other. The critical issue for the estimation of panel data models is whether the individual effects μ_i are correlated with the observed regressors X. Failure to account for correlation between μ_i and X in estimating the panel data regression model leads to inconsistent estimates of the slope coefficients, β.

TABLE 13 - LINEAR RANDOM EFFECTS MODEL (GLS)

```
Random-effects GLS regression              Number of obs      =      4342
Group variable (i) : serno                 Number of groups   =      3062

R-sq:  within  = 0.0535                     Obs per group: min =         1
       between = 0.0966                                    avg =       1.4
       overall = 0.0911                                    max =         2

Random effects u_i ~ Gaussian               Wald chi2(27)     =    396.57
corr(u_i, X)       = 0 (assumed)            Prob > chi2       =    0.0000
```

yvar	Coef.	Std. Err.	z	P>|z|	[95% Conf. Interval]	
male	2.898659	.3396536	8.53	0.000	2.23295	3.564368
age	-.0304106	.0215193	-1.41	0.158	-.0725876	.0117664
age2	-.6439257	.0761712	-8.45	0.000	-.7932185	-.4946329
age3	.5998144	.2800377	2.14	0.032	.0509507	1.148678
ethbawi	-5.859856	1.596165	-3.67	0.000	-8.988283	-2.73143
ethipb	-4.795425	1.43272	-3.35	0.001	-7.603505	-1.987344
ethothnw	-3.686484	1.686421	-2.19	0.029	-6.991809	-.3811602
part	-.8124215	.415153	-1.96	0.050	-1.626106	.0012634
unemp	-1.013121	.4948661	-2.05	0.041	-1.983041	-.0432012
retd	-1.520195	.5347246	-2.84	0.004	-2.568235	-.4721536
stdnt	.183426	1.542036	0.12	0.905	-2.838909	3.205761
keephse	-.4214062	.4262893	-0.99	0.323	-1.256918	.4141055
lsch14u	2.081061	.975074	2.13	0.033	.1699509	3.992171
lsch14	.5854126	.558657	1.05	0.295	-.5095351	1.68036
lsch15	1.140985	.4170894	2.74	0.006	.3235052	1.958466
lsch17	.235464	.6325691	0.37	0.710	-1.004349	1.475277
lsch18	-.9055674	.7327179	-1.24	0.216	-2.341668	.5305333
lsch19	-2.69433	1.582058	-1.70	0.089	-5.795106	.406446
regsc1s	.4088833	.8065552	0.51	0.612	-1.171936	1.989702
regsc2	.1463989	.3887129	0.38	0.706	-.6154643	.9082621
regsc3n	-.8087709	.4412171	-1.83	0.067	-1.673541	.0559988
regsc4	-.0969798	.3478152	-0.28	0.780	-.7786852	.5847255
regsc5n	.7526405	.4842886	1.55	0.120	-.1965477	1.701829
widow	1.030657	.59798	1.72	0.085	-.1413624	2.202676
single	.017102	.4613643	0.04	0.970	-.8871553	.9213594
seprd	3.444529	.6674898	5.16	0.000	2.136273	4.752785
divorce	.7209378	.5041313	1.43	0.153	-.2671413	1.709017
_cons	16.18108	.48061	33.67	0.000	15.23911	17.12306
sigma_u	6.5221676					
sigma_e	5.4933769					
rho	.58499852	(fraction of variance due to u_i)				

The presence of a common individual effect means that the values of the dependent variable for each individual will tend to cluster together. This clustering can be allowed for using the **generalised least squares estimator (GLS)** which allows for the fact that an error term for a particular individual will be correlated over the waves of the panel. However, use of the GLS estimator assumes that the individual effect is uncorrelated with the explanatory variables X. This problem can be dealt with by using deviations to sweep the unobservable individual effect out of the equation. One way of doing this is to take *mean deviations*, measuring each variable as the deviation from the within-individual mean of the variables. Alternatively the variables can be measured as *first differences*, by subtracting the value in period t-1 from the value in period t. Because the individual effect is assumed to be constant over time, taking deviations eliminates μ from the equation. Applying the standard least squares estimator to the transformed variables gives the *covariance* or *within-groups estimator* of ß, which is **consistent** even when the individual effect is correlated with the explanatory variables. However, for this estimator to work in practice, there must be sufficient within-individual variability in the dependent variable and the explanatory variables. The estimator will tend not to work well in a short panel (where T is small) and where there is not much variation within groups. These problems go away when the group size is large, in other words when T is large. In that case the GLS or random effects estimator can be shown to be equivalent to the within-groups or fixed effects estimator (see Blundell and Windmeijer, 1997).

The **random effects** and **fixed effects** estimators for the linear panel data model are illustrated using data on the number of cigarettes smoked per day for the sub-sample of smokers in the HALS data. Table 13 shows the random effects GLS regression and Table 14 shows the fixed effects within-groups regression. The models are estimated using the two waves of the HALS data. As some individuals who took part in the first survey did not respond to, or could not be traced for, the second survey, the models are estimated on the **unbalanced panel**, using all available observations on the dependent variable. This means that more data are included for individuals at wave 1 than at wave 2.

In the GLS model, the error components specification means that the overall variance of the error term can be decomposed into two components, σ^2_μ associated with the individual effect and σ^2_μ associated with the idiosyncratic error term. Table 13 gives estimates of σ_μ (sigma_u) and σ_ϵ (sigma_e) and also reports the value of ρ, the

TABLE 14 - LINEAR FIXED EFFECTS MODEL

```
Fixed-effects (within) regression          Number of obs     =      4342
Group variable (i) : serno                 Number of groups  =      3062

R-sq:  within  = 0.0648                     Obs per group: min =         1
       between = 0.0341                                    avg =       1.4
       overall = 0.0362                                    max =         2

                                            F(17,1263)        =      5.15
corr(u_i, Xb)  = -0.0951                     Prob > F          =    0.0000
```

yvar	Coef.	Std. Err.	t	P>|t|	[95% Conf. Interval]
male	(dropped)					
age	-.0413616	.0449158	-0.92	0.357	-.1294795	.0467562
age2	-.8270015	.1331349	-6.21	0.000	-1.088191	-.5658115
age3	.2895262	.4886271	0.59	0.554	-.669084	1.248136
ethbawi	(dropped)					
ethipb	(dropped)					
ethothnw	(dropped)					
part	-.3915503	.5977959	-0.65	0.513	-1.564333	.781232
unemp	-3.055652	.787098	-3.88	0.000	-4.599815	-1.511488
retd	-.6765088	.7617225	-0.89	0.375	-2.170889	.8178718
stdnt	1.680867	2.361335	0.71	0.477	-2.951703	6.313437
keephse	-.4300261	.6682942	-0.64	0.520	-1.741115	.881063
lsch14u	(dropped)					
lsch14	(dropped)					
lsch15	(dropped)					
lsch17	(dropped)					
lsch18	(dropped)					
lsch19	(dropped)					
regsc1s	.2942756	1.379834	0.21	0.831	-2.412744	3.001295
regsc2	.2913165	.7241938	0.40	0.688	-1.129439	1.712072
regsc3n	.4087132	.8046426	0.51	0.612	-1.16987	1.987296
regsc4	-.1300566	.5771256	-0.23	0.822	-1.262287	1.002174
regsc5n	1.211408	.8220318	1.47	0.141	-.40129	2.824106
widow	1.832758	1.188608	1.54	0.123	-.4991061	4.164622
single	.3852976	1.038784	0.37	0.711	-1.652634	2.42323
seprd	3.020071	.9732749	3.10	0.002	1.110658	4.929485
divorce	.1297901	.8413171	0.15	0.877	-1.520743	1.780323
_cons	18.23225	.4476278	40.73	0.000	17.35407	19.11042

```
sigma_u |  8.4461331
sigma_e |  5.4933769
    rho |   .70272983   (fraction of variance due to u_i)
```

```
F test that all u_i=0:     F(3061, 1263) =      2.96          Prob > F = 0.0000
```

intra-group correlation coefficient, which has a value of 0.585. This shows the fraction of the overall variance of the error term that can be attributed to the individual effect. The coefficients of the regression function can be interpreted in the usual way. They show, for example, that individuals with more years of schooling smoke fewer cigarettes and those with fewer years of formal schooling smoke more.

As it only has two waves, the HALS data are not well-suited to the fixed effects estimator, particularly as the two waves are seven years apart. In applying the within-groups estimator, any time invariant variables, such as the individual's gender or ethnic group are eliminated from the regression. The remaining variables are measured as deviations from the within-individual mean. Table 14 is included only for comparison with the random effects estimates. The fact that HALS only has two waves means that the within-groups estimator performs very poorly. The method would come into its own with a longer panel, providing more information on each individual's behaviour as it evolves over time.

TABLE 15 - POOLED PROBIT MODEL

```
Probit estimates                           Number of obs   =      14209
                                           LR chi2(27)     =     702.71
                                           Prob > chi2     =     0.0000
Log likelihood = -7989.9167                Pseudo R2       =     0.0421
```

yvar	Coef.	Std. Err.	z	P>|z|	[95% Conf.	Interval]
male	-.0068974	.0273188	-0.25	0.801	-.0604412	.0466464
age	-.0064117	.0017746	-3.61	0.000	-.0098898	-.0029336
age2	-.0332207	.0071209	-4.67	0.000	-.0471774	-.0192641
age3	.1101963	.0215749	5.11	0.000	.0679102	.1524823
ethbawi	-.2863132	.1133627	-2.53	0.012	-.5085	-.0641265
ethipb	-.3594183	.0983905	-3.65	0.000	-.5522602	-.1665764
ethothnw	-.3499534	.1367414	-2.56	0.010	-.6179616	-.0819452
part	.1555199	.0413251	3.76	0.000	.0745242	.2365156
unemp	-.138589	.0571241	-2.43	0.015	-.2505502	-.0266278
retd	-.0461887	.0497158	-0.93	0.353	-.1436298	.0512524
stdnt	.1145091	.1323305	0.87	0.387	-.1448538	.373872
keephse	-.1218374	.0420513	-2.90	0.004	-.2042565	-.0394184
lsch14u	-.3097408	.0689802	-4.49	0.000	-.4449396	-.1745421
lsch14	-.2626227	.0416924	-6.30	0.000	-.3443383	-.180907
lsch15	-.1576634	.0342902	-4.60	0.000	-.224871	-.0904559
lsch17	.0802489	.0481798	1.67	0.096	-.0141818	.1746796
lsch18	.1988208	.0512741	3.88	0.000	.0983254	.2993162
lsch19	-.0052156	.1063857	-0.05	0.961	-.2137278	.2032966
regsc1s	.3506734	.0604204	5.80	0.000	.2322516	.4690951
regsc2	.2177603	.0333292	6.53	0.000	.1524362	.2830843
regsc3n	.0920397	.0376473	2.44	0.014	.0182524	.165827
regsc4	-.0802458	.0333909	-2.40	0.016	-.1456907	-.0148009
regsc5n	-.2028511	.0484185	-4.19	0.000	-.2977497	-.1079526
widow	-.1249198	.0439715	-2.84	0.004	-.2111024	-.0387373
single	-.1134637	.0408279	-2.78	0.005	-.1934849	-.0334425
seprd	-.2058863	.0787671	-2.61	0.009	-.3602671	-.0515056
divorce	-.1783488	.0549352	-3.25	0.001	-.2860199	-.0706777
_cons	.8050736	.0410885	19.59	0.000	.7245416	.8856057

10.2 Binary choices

The discussion so far has concentrated on a simple linear panel data regression model in which the dependent variable can take a continuous range of values. In practice, analysts using health surveys are more likely to be confronted with qualitative or categorical dependent variables. These make estimation of panel data models more complex. The linear specification is attractive because taking differences or mean deviations allows the individual effect to be swept from the equation. But this is no longer possible for a non-linear regression model as typically used for qualitative and categorical variables. To illustrate, consider a binary choice model,

$$E(y|X_{it}\beta, \mu_i) = P(y_i=1|X_{it}\beta, \mu_i) = F(X_{it}\beta + \mu_i) \tag{12}$$

Taking differences or mean deviations of the non-linear function F(.) will not eliminate the individual effect. This is a problem if the individual effects are expected to be correlated with the explanatory variables.

If an analyst is willing to assume that the effects and the explanatory variables are uncorrelated, then the clustering of the dependent variable can be dealt with using a random effects specification. For example, the **random effects probit** model assumes that both components of the error term are normally distributed and that both are independent of the X_{it}. By assuming a specific distribution for the individual effect it is possible to write down a sample log likelihood function that allows for the correlation in the error term within individuals. This expression can be estimated using standard software, such as Stata.

Let us return to the example of the binary measure of self-assessed health, where y equals 1 if an individual reports 'excellent' or 'good' health and equals 0 if an individual reports 'fair' or 'poor' health. Now we can make use of the longitudinal element of HALS and use information from both waves of the survey. The first set of estimates, presented in Table 15, are for a *pooled probit* specification. This simply takes the standard **probit** estimator and ignores the fact that we are dealing with repeated observations. It pools all of the observations together, not allowing for the fact that some individuals are measured twice. This means that the model is estimated on the basis of a wrongly specified likelihood function. However, it can be shown that the estimator does give **consistent** estimates of the ß's, even though it ignores the structure of the error term. Compare these estimates with

TABLE 16 - RANDOM EFFECTS PROBIT MODEL

```
Random-effects probit                         Number of obs      =       14209
Group variable (i) : serno                    Number of groups   =        8952

Random effects u_i ~ Gaussian                 Obs per group: min =           1
                                                             avg =         1.6
                                                             max =           2

                                              Wald chi2(27)      =      468.39
Log likelihood  = -7734.4866                  Prob > chi2        =      0.0000
```

yvar	Coef.	Std. Err.	z	P>|z|	[95% Conf.	Interval]
male	-.0137224	.0429172	-0.32	0.749	-.0978385	.0703937
age	-.0069471	.002674	-2.60	0.009	-.012188	-.0017062
age2	-.0559292	.0105351	-5.31	0.000	-.0765777	-.0352807
age3	.1467533	.0317494	4.62	0.000	.0845256	.208981
ethbawi	-.4072376	.179303	-2.27	0.023	-.758665	-.0558103
ethipb	-.5340048	.1548172	-3.45	0.001	-.8374409	-.2305687
ethothnw	-.5189814	.218082	-2.38	0.017	-.9464143	-.0915485
part	.1804717	.0597389	3.02	0.003	.0633855	.2975578
unemp	-.1318259	.0820375	-1.61	0.108	-.2926165	.0289646
retd	-.0619076	.070894	-0.87	0.383	-.2008572	.077042
stdnt	.1960319	.189486	1.03	0.301	-.1753538	.5674175
keephse	-.1359808	.061703	-2.20	0.028	-.2569165	-.0150451
lsch14u	-.4855768	.1103036	-4.40	0.000	-.701768	-.2693857
lsch14	-.4201722	.067375	-6.24	0.000	-.5522247	-.2881197
lsch15	-.2370722	.0552643	-4.29	0.000	-.3453882	-.1287562
lsch17	.1265407	.0771395	1.64	0.101	-.02465	.2777315
lsch18	.3343847	.0825078	4.05	0.000	.1726724	.4960971
lsch19	.007423	.1705596	0.04	0.965	-.3268677	.3417137
regsc1s	.444602	.091641	4.85	0.000	.2649889	.6242151
regsc2	.2700588	.0511486	5.28	0.000	.1698094	.3703082
regsc3n	.0773983	.0570371	1.36	0.175	-.0343925	.1891891
regsc4	-.1157136	.0502118	-2.30	0.021	-.214127	-.0173003
regsc5n	-.2983758	.0728549	-4.10	0.000	-.4411687	-.1555829
widow	-.1646477	.066808	-2.46	0.014	-.2955891	-.0337064
single	-.1199239	.0627868	-1.91	0.056	-.2429838	.0031359
seprd	-.2844771	.1121935	-2.54	0.011	-.5043724	-.0645818
divorce	-.2407617	.0822965	-2.93	0.003	-.4020599	-.0794635
_cons	1.207721	.0687456	17.57	0.000	1.072982	1.34246
/lnsig2u	.1289803	.0800067			-.02783	.2857907
sigma_u	1.066615	.0426682			.9861814	1.153609
rho	.5322005	.0199187			.493043	.5709653

```
Likelihood ratio test of rho=0: chibar2(01) =   510.86 Prob >= chibar2 = 0.000
```

the cross-section results for the probit model in Table 2. Now we have a larger sample because we are using information from wave 2 as well as wave 1. Again, the ß coefficients should be interpreted as qualitative effects and quantitative inferences should be made on the basis of average or marginal effects. Once more, we can see clear gradients in self-assessed health by education and by occupational socio-economic group.

Table 16 shows the random effects probit model. The table includes an estimate of ρ, the intra-group correlation coefficient. This suggests that the individual effect accounts for around half (0.532) of the random variation.

Recall that the random effects probit model embodies two important assumptions: that the individual effect has a normal distribution and that it is uncorrelated with the explanatory variables. The first assumption can be relaxed by using a **semiparametric** approach. For example, Deb (2001) develops a finite mixture random effects probit model, using the same sort of methods that were described in the sections on health data and duration models.

The second assumption – that the individual effects are uncorrelated with the explanatory variables – can be dealt with in two ways. The first is to adopt a fixed effects specification, treating the individual effects as parameters to be estimated, or at least eliminated from the model. The second is to use a *correlated random effects* specification.

It has already been stressed that, for most non-linear models, the convenient device for taking mean deviations or first differences is no longer feasible. This is certainly the case for the panel data probit model. However, the logit model is an exception to this rule. Because of the special features of the logistic function, it is possible to re-formulate the model in a way that eliminates the individual effect, μ. By restricting attention to those individuals who change status during the course of the panel, it is possible to estimate the standard logit model using first differences in the explanatory variables, rather than the levels of the variables. This means that the standard logit model can be applied to differenced data and the individual effect is swept out in the process. Like the fixed effects estimator for linear models, this approach will work well only if there is sufficient within-individual variation in the variables.

Another approach to dealing with individual random effects that are correlated with the explanatory variables is to specify this relationship directly. For example, in dealing with the random effects probit model, Chamberlain (1984) suggested specifying this relationship as a linear regression of the value of the explanatory variables in all of the waves of the panel. This function is then substituted back into the original equation and, as long as there is sufficient within-individual variation, it allows separate estimates of the ß's and of the correlation between the X's and the individual effect to be disentangled (see the Technical Appendix and Jones, 2000, for details of this method). In this sense, this method has a strong parallel with the within-group estimator.

11 Concluding Thoughts

This booklet has illustrated the diversity of applied econometric methods that are available to health economists who work with microdata. The text has emphasised the range of models and estimators that are available, but that should not imply a neglect of the need for sound economic theory and careful data collection to produce worthwhile econometric research. Most of the methods reviewed here are designed for individual level data. Because of the widespread use of observational data in health economics, particular care should be devoted to dealing with problems of self-selection and unobservable heterogeneity. This is likely to set the agenda for future research, with the emphasis on robust estimators applied to panel data and other complex datasets.

References

Blundell, R.W. and F.A.G. Windmeijer (1997), 'Correlated cluster effects and simultaneity in multilevel models', *Health Economics* **6**: 439-443.

Chamberlain, G. (1984), 'Panel data' in Griliches, Z. and M. Intrilligator, eds., *North-Holland handbook of econometrics* (Elsevier, Amsterdam): 1247-1318.

Cox, B.D. et al. (1987), *The Health and Lifestyle Survey*, The Health Promotion Research Trust.

Cox, B.D., F.A. Huppert and M.J. Whichelow (1993), *The Health and Lifestyle Survey: seven years on,* (Dartmouth, Aldershot).

Deb, P. (2001), 'A discrete random effects probit model with application to the demand for preventive care', *Health Economics* **10**: 371-383.

Deb, P. and P.K. Trivedi (1997), 'Demand for medical care by the elderly: a finite mixture approach', *Journal of Applied Econometrics* **12**: 313-336.

Forster, M. and Jones, A.M. (2001), 'The role of taxes in starting and quitting smoking: duration analysis of British data', *Journal of the Royal Statistical Society (Series A)*, **164**: 517-547.

Heckman, J.J. (1979), 'Sample selection bias as a specification error', *Econometrica* **47**: 153-161.

Heckman, J.J. and B. Singer (1984), 'A method of minimizing the distributional impact in econometric models for duration data', *Econometrica* **52**: 271-230.

Jones, A.M. (2000), 'Health econometrics', in *North-Holland handbook of health economics*, A.J. Culyer and J.P. Newhouse (eds.), (Elsevier, Amsterdam), pp.265-344, 2000.

Kiefer, N. (1988), 'Economic duration data and hazard functions', *Journal of Economic Literature* **26**: 646-679.

Leung, S.F. and S. Yu (1996), 'On the choice between sample selection and two-part models', *Journal of Econometrics* **72**: 197-229.

Mullahy, J. (1997), 'Heterogeneity, excess zeros, and the structure of count data models', *Journal of Applied Econometrics* **12**: 337-350.

Suggested Further Reading

General:

Deaton, A. (1997), *The analysis of household surveys: a microeconometric approach to development policy,* published for the World Bank by Johns Hopkins University Press.

Greene, W.H. (2000), *Econometric analysis*, Prentice Hall.

Jones, A.M. (2000), 'Health econometrics', in *North-Holland handbook of health economics*, A.J. Culyer and J.P. Newhouse (eds.), (Elsevier, Amsterdam), pp.265-344, 2000.

Verbeek, M. (2000), *Modern econometrics,* Wiley.

Qualitative dependent variables:

Gourieroux, C. (2000), *Econometrics of qualitative dependent variables*, Cambridge University Press.

Maddala, G.S. (1983), *Limited dependent and qualitative variables in econometrics*, Cambridge University Press.

Pudney, S. (1989), *Modelling individual choice: the econometrics of corners, kinks and holes*, Blackwell.

Sample selection:

Vella, F. (1998), 'Estimating models with sample selection bias', *Journal of Human Resources* **33**: 127-169.

Count data:

Cameron, A.C. and P.K. Trivedi (1998), *Regression analysis of count data*, Cambridge University Press.

Duration analysis:

Lancaster, T. (1992), *The econometric analysis of transition data*, Cambridge University Press.

Panel data:

Baltagi, B.H. (2001), *Econometric analysis of panel data, 2nd edition*, Wiley.

Glossary

Asymptotic property: A property of a statistic that applies as the sample size grows large (specifically, as it tends to infinity).

Attrition bias: Bias caused by unit non-response in panel data. This occurs when the individuals who drop out of a panel study are systematically different from those who remain in a panel study.

Average effect: A measure of the effect of a binary explanatory variable, X, on the outcome of interest; based on comparing the outcome when X equals 1 with the outcome when X equals 0.

Binary variable: A variable that takes only two values, usually coded as zero and one.

Bivariate probit model: A model that combines two binary probit models to deal with a system of two binary dependent variables.

Consistent estimate: An estimate that converges on the true parameter value as the sample size increases (towards infinity).

Continuous variable: A variable that can take the value of any real number within an interval.

Cox proportional hazard model: A semiparametric model for duration analysis.

Cross-section data: Survey data in which each respondent is observed only once, giving a 'snapshot' view of the population at a point in time.

Dummy variable: Another label for binary variables that take the value zero or one.

Error components model: A regression model for panel data.

Excess zeros: A feature of count data, when the number of zeroes observed exceeds the number that would be expected from the Poisson model.

Fixed effects: The fixed effects specification treats the individual effects in panel data models as parameters to be estimated. This is appropriate when inferences are to be confined to the effects in the sample only, and the effects themselves are of substantive interest (see **random effects**).

Gamma distribution: Probability distribution often used to model individual heterogeneity, especially in count data regression and duration analysis.

GMM: Many of the estimators discussed in this booklet fall within the unifying framework of generalised method of moments (GMM) estimation. This replaces population moment conditions (e.g. based on expected values) with their sample analogues (e.g. based on sample means).

Generalized least squares (GLS): A generalization of **ordinary least squares** which relaxes the assumption that the error terms are independently and identically distributed across observations.

Grouped data regression: See **interval regression**.

Heckit model: A two-step estimator designed to deal with the **sample selection** problem.

Heteroscedasticity: When the variance of the error term is not constant across observations.

Homoscedasticity: When the variance of the error term is constant across observations.

Instrumental variables: A method of estimation for models with endogenous regressors – regressors that are correlated with the error term. It relies on variables (or 'instruments') that are good predictors of an endogenous regressor, but are not independently related to the dependent variable. These may be used to purge the bias caused by endogeneity.

Interval regression: A variant on the ordered probit model that can be used when the threshold values are known.

Inverse Mill's ratio (IMR): The label given to the hazard rate (ratio of density to survival functions) for a **probit model**. The IMR can be interpreted as the (generalised) residual of the probit model and it is used in the **Heckit** correction for sample selection bias.

Item non-response: When a respondent does not provide data for a particular variable in a survey.

Linear probability model: A model for binary dependent variables based on the linear regression model.

Logistic distribution: A continuous probability distribution that is the foundation for the **logit** model of binary choice.

Logit: A model for binary dependent variables based on the **logistic distribution**.

Marginal effect: A measure of the effect of a continuous explanatory variable, X, on the outcome of interest; based on the derivative of the outcome with respect to X.

Maximum likelihood estimation: A method of estimation that specifies the joint probability of the observed set of data and finds the parameter values that maximize it (i.e. that are most likely).

Multinomial logit model: A model for unordered multinomial outcomes.

Negbin model: An extension of the Poisson regression model for count data.

Normal distribution: A continuous probability distribution that has a typical 'bell-shape'. Used as the foundation for classical regression and analysis and many other models such as the **probit model** and the **Heckit model**.

Ordered probit model: A model for ordered multinomial outcomes.

Ordinary least squares (OLS): The standard method for fitting the classical linear regression model. It is based on finding the parameter values that minimize the sum of squared errors.

Over-dispersion: When observed count data is more spread out than would be expected from a Poisson model.

Panel data: Survey data in which each respondent is observed repeatedly over time.

Point estimate: A single number used to estimate an unknown parameter (the 'best guess'). As opposed to an interval estimate, which presents a range of values.

Poisson regression: A model for count data.

Probit model: A model for binary dependent variables based on the standard **normal distribution**.

Qualitative effect: The sign of the effect of one variable on another.

Quantitative effect: The magnitude of the effect of one variable on another.

Random effects: The random effects specification treats the individual effects in panel data models as random draws. If individual effects are not of intrinsic importance in themselves, and are assumed to be random draws from a population of individuals, and if inferences concerning population effects and their characteristics are sought, then a random specification is suitable (see **fixed effects**).

Random effects probit: A model for binary dependent variables in panel data.

RESET: A general test for mis-specification of the functional form of a regression model and for omitted variables.

SAH: Self-assessed health status.

Sample selection bias: The bias created when non-responders are systematically different from responders.

Semiparametric: A method that mixes parametric assumptions (e.g. that the relationship between y and X is linear) and non-parametric assumptions (e.g. that the distribution of the error term is unknown).

Unit non-response: When a potential respondent does not provide data for any variables in a survey.

Unbalanced panel: A panel dataset that includes all respondents who report data for at least one period (wave) of the panel. In contrast to a balanced panel which only includes those individuals with complete data for all periods.

Weibull model: A parametric model for duration analysis.

Weighted least squares: Weights (w_i) are attached to the values of the dependent variable (y_i) and independent variables (X_i) before using least squares regression. This method can be used to correct for heteroscedasticity.

Technical Appendix

1. Binary responses

When y equals 0 or 1, the conditional expectation of y is:

$$E(y_i|x_i) = P(y_i=1|x_i) = F(x_i) \tag{A1}$$

The most common nonlinear parametric specifications are logit and probit models. These can be given a latent variable interpretation. Let:

$$y_i = 1 \quad \text{iff } y^*_i > 0 \tag{A2}$$
$$= 0 \quad \text{otherwise}$$

where,

$$y^*_i = x_i\beta + \epsilon_i$$

Then,

$$P(y_i=1| x_i) = P(y^*_i >0| x_i) = P(\epsilon_i >-x_i\beta) = F(x_i\beta) \tag{A3}$$

The log-likelihood for a sample of independent observations is,

$$\text{LogL} = \Sigma_i \{(1-y_i)\log(1-F(x_i\beta)) + y_i \log(F(x_i\beta))\} \tag{A4}$$

2. Multinomial and ordered responses

Ordered probit

The ordered probit model can be used to model a discrete dependent variable that takes ordered multinomial outcomes, e.g. $y = 1,2......,m$.

$$y_i = j \text{ if } \mu_{j-1} < y^*_i \leq \mu_j , j = 1,......m \tag{A5}$$

where,

$$y^*_i = x_i\beta + \epsilon_i , \epsilon_i \sim N(0,1) \tag{A6}$$

and $\mu_0 = -\infty$, $\mu_j \leq \mu_{j+1}$, $\mu_m = \infty$.

$$P_{ij} = P(y_i = j) = \Phi(\mu_j - x_i\beta) - \Phi(\mu_{j-1} - x_i\beta) \tag{A7}$$

The log-likelihood takes the form,

$$\text{LogL} = \Sigma_i \, \Sigma_j \, y_{ij} \, \log P_{ij} \qquad \text{(A8)}$$

where y_{ij} is a binary variable that equals 1 if $y_i = j$.

Multinomial logit

Multinomial models apply to discrete dependent variables that can take (unordered) multinomial outcomes, $y = 1,2,\ldots,m$. Define a set of binary variables to indicate which alternative ($j = 1,\ldots,m$) is chosen by each individual ($i = 1,\ldots,n$),

$$\begin{aligned} y_{ij} &= 1 \quad \text{if } y_i = j \\ &= 0 \quad \text{otherwise} \end{aligned} \qquad \text{(A9)}$$

with associated probabilities,

$$P(y_i = j) = P_{ij} \qquad \text{(A10)}$$

With independent observations, the log-likelihood for a multinomial model takes the form,

$$\text{LogL} = \Sigma_i \, \Sigma_j \, y_{ij} \, \log P_{ij} \qquad \text{(A11)}$$

The multinomial logit model uses,

$$P_{ij} = \exp(x_i \beta_j) \, / \, \Sigma_k \exp(x_i \beta_k) \qquad \text{(A12)}$$

with a normalisation that $\beta_m = 0$.

Bivariate probit

The bivariate probit model applies to a pair of binary dependent variables,

$$y^*_{ji} = x_{ji}\beta_j + \epsilon_j, \, j = 1,2, \, (\epsilon_1,\epsilon_2) \sim N(0,\Omega) \qquad \text{(A13)}$$

where,

$$\begin{aligned} y_{ji} &= 1 \quad \text{iff } y^*_{ji} > 0 \\ &= 0 \quad \text{otherwise} \end{aligned} \qquad \text{(A14)}$$

3. The sample selection model

It is possible to express the sample selection model in terms of latent variables (y^*),

$$y^*_{ji} = x_{ji}\beta_j + \epsilon_j \, , \, j = 1,2 \qquad (A15)$$

Then the sample selection model is given by,

$$y_i = y^*_{2i} \quad \text{iff } y^*_{1i} > 0 \qquad (A16)$$
$$= \text{unobserved otherwise}$$

4. Count data regression

The Poisson process

$$P(y_i) = e^{-\lambda_i}\lambda_i^{y_i} / y_i! \qquad (A17)$$

This gives the probability of observing a count of y_i events during a fixed interval. In order to condition the outcome (y) on a set of regressors (x), it is usually assumed that,

$$\lambda_i = E(y_i|x_i) = \exp(x_i\beta) \qquad (A18)$$

An important feature of the Poisson model is the equidispersion property, that

$$E(y_i|x_i) = \text{Var}(y_i|x_i) = \lambda_i.$$

Maximum likelihood estimation (ML) uses the fully specified probability distribution and maximises the log-likelihood,

$$\text{LogL} = \Sigma_i \log[P(y_i)] \qquad (A19)$$

The first-order moment condition implies an alternative formulation of the Poisson model, as a nonlinear regression equation,

$$E(y_i|x_i) = \exp(x_i\beta) \qquad (A20)$$

Overdispersion and the negbin model

The negative binomial specification allows for overdispersion by specifying,

$$\exp(x_i\beta + \mu_i) = [\exp(x_i\beta)]\eta_i$$

where η_i is a gamma distributed error term. Then,

$$P(y_i) = \{\Gamma(y_i+\psi_i)/\Gamma(\psi_i)\Gamma(y_i+1)\}(\psi_i/(\lambda_i+\psi_i))^{\psi_i}(\lambda_i/(\lambda_i+\psi_i))^{y_i} \qquad (A21)$$

where $\Gamma(.)$ is the gamma function. Letting the 'precision parameter' $\psi = (1/a)\lambda^k$, for $a > 0$, gives,

$$E(y) = \lambda \text{ and } Var(y) = \lambda + a\lambda^{2-k} \qquad (A22)$$

This leads to two special cases: setting $k = 1$ gives the negbin 1 model with the variance proportional to the mean, $(1 + a)\lambda$; and setting $k = 0$ gives the negbin 2 model where the variance is a quadratic function of the mean, $\lambda + a\lambda^2$. Setting $a = 0$ gives the Poisson model, and this nesting can be tested using a conventional t-test.

The 'zero-inflated' or 'with zeros' model

The probability function for the zero inflated Poisson model, $P^{ZIP}(y|x)$ is related to the standard Poisson model, $P^P(y|x)$, as follows:

$$P^{ZIP}(y|x) = 1(y=0)q + (1-q)P^P(y|x) \qquad (A23)$$

where $1(y=0)$ is an indicator function which takes the value 1 if $y = 0$, and takes the value 0 otherwise.

Hurdle/two-part specifications

The hurdle model assumes that the participation decision and the positive count are generated by separate probability processes $P_1(.)$ and $P_2(.)$. The log-likelihood for the hurdle model is,

$$LogL = \Sigma_{y=0} \log[1-P_1(y>0|x)] + \Sigma_{y>0} \{\log[P_1(y>0|x)] + \log[P_2(y|x,y>0)]\}$$

$$= \{\Sigma_{y=0} \log[1-P_1(y>0|x)] + \Sigma_{y>0} \log[P_1(y>0|x)]\} + \{\Sigma_{y>0} \log[P_2(y|x,y>0)]\}$$

$$= LogL_1 + LogL_2 \qquad (A24)$$

This shows that the two parts of the model can be estimated separately; with a binary process ($LogL_1$) and the truncated at zero count model ($LogL_2$).

Finite mixture approach

The model is implemented using a finite density estimator, where each population, j, is represented by a probability mass point, p_j, (see Heckman and Singer, 1984). The C-point finite mixture negbin model takes the form,

$$P(y_i|.) = \Sigma^C_{j=1} \, p_j.P_j(y_i|.), \; \Sigma^C_{j=1} \, p_j = 1 \; , \; 0 \leq p_j \leq 1 \qquad (A25)$$

where each of the $P_j(y_i|.)$ is a separate negbin model, and the p_j's are estimated along with the other parameters of the model.

5. Duration analysis

Semiparametric models

In the Cox model, the hazard function at time t for individual i, $h_i(t, x_i)$, is defined as the product of a baseline hazard function, $h_0(t)$, and a proportionality factor, $\exp(x_i\beta)$,

$$h_i(t, x_i) = h_0(t).\exp(x_i\beta) \qquad (A26)$$

where x_i is a vector of covariates and β is a parameter vector.

Parametric models

Specifying the baseline hazard function as $h_0(t) = hpt^{p-1}$ gives the Weibull proportional hazards model,

$$h_i(t) = hpt^{p-1}.\exp(x_i\beta) \qquad (A27)$$

where p is known as the shape parameter. The hazard is monotonically increasing for p>1, showing increasing duration dependence, and monotonically decreasing for p<1, showing decreasing duration dependence.

The hazard function, $h(t)=f(t)/S(t)$, can be used to derive the probability density function, $f(t)$, and the survival function, $S(t)$, for the Weibull model. The likelihood function with right censoring is,

$$L = \Pi_i \, \{f_i(t)/S_i(t)\}^{\delta i} .S_i(t) \qquad (A28)$$

Unobservable heterogeneity

Kiefer (1988) shows how unobservable heterogeneity can be incorporated by adding a general heterogeneity effect μ and specifying,

$$f(t) = \int f(t|\mu)p(\mu)d\mu \tag{A29}$$

The unknown distribution $p(\mu)$ can be modelled parametrically using mixture distributions. Alternatively a non-parametric approach can be adopted which gives μ a discrete distribution characterised by the mass-points,

$$P(\mu=\mu_i) = p_i , \; i = 1,......,I \tag{A30}$$

where the parameters $(\mu_1,......, \mu_n, p_1,......, p_n)$ are estimated as part of the maximum likelihood estimation. This is the basis for the finite support density estimator of Heckman and Singer (1984).

6. Longitudinal and hierarchical data

Linear models

The standard linear panel data regression model, in which there are repeated measurements $(t=1,...., T)$ for a sample of n individuals $(i=1,.....,n)$, is:

$$y_{it} = x_{it}\beta + \mu_i + \epsilon_{it} \tag{A31}$$

Binary choice

Now consider a nonlinear model, for example a binary choice model based on the latent variable specification,

$$y^*_{it} = x_{it}\beta + \mu_i + \epsilon_{it}, \text{ where } y_{it} = 1 \text{ if } y^*_{it} > 0, \; 0 \text{ otherwise.} \tag{A32}$$

Then, assuming that the distribution of ϵ_{it} is symmetric with distribution function F(.),

$$P(y_{it} = 1) = P(\epsilon_{it} > -x_{it}\beta - \mu_i) = F(x_{it}\beta + \mu_i) \tag{A33}$$

The conditional logit

The conditional logit estimator uses the fact that $\Sigma_t y_{it}$ is a sufficient statistic for μ_i. Using the logistic function,

$$P(y_{it} = 1) = F(x_{it}\beta + \mu_i) = exp(x_{it}\beta + \mu_i)/(1 + exp(x_{it}\beta + \mu_i)) \qquad (A34)$$

it is possible to show that,

$$P[(0,1)|(0,1) \text{ or } (1,0)] = exp((x_{i2} - x_{i1})\beta)/(1 + exp((x_{i2} - x_{i1})\beta)) \qquad (A35)$$

In other words, the standard logit model can be applied to differenced data and the individual effect is swept out.

Parameterising the individual effect

Another approach to dealing with individual effects that are correlated with the regressors is to specify $E(\mu|x)$ directly, for example:

$$\mu_i = x_i\alpha + u_i, \ u_i \sim iid \ N(0, \sigma^2) \qquad (A36)$$

where $x_i = (x_{i1},....,x_{iT})$. Then, for the random effects probit model the distribution of y_{it} conditional on x but marginal to μ_i has the probit form,

$$P(y_{it} = 1) = \Phi[(1 + \sigma^2)^{-1/2}(x_{it}\beta + x_i\alpha)] \qquad (A37)$$

Stata Code Appendix

```
* This is the program to estimate the models described in this booklet
* using Stata Version 7. The code is written in a general format with
* the dependent variables called yvar (created using "gen yvar = ......")
* and the list of independent variables called $xvars (created using
* "global xvars "male age...."") . The estimation sample for each model
*  is selected using the "if" command e.g., observations from the
*  first wave of HALS are selected by "if wave==1".

*********** BINARY CHOICE MODELS *************;

* LINEAR PROBABILITY MODEL;

regress yvar $xvars if wave==1;

* RESET test;
predict yf, xb;
gen yf2=yf^2;
quietly regress yvar $xvars yf2 if wave==1;
test yf2=0;

* WEIGHTED LEAST SQUARES TO ALLOW FOR HETEROSKEDASTICITY;
gen wt=yf*(1-yf);
regress yvar $xvars [aweight=wt] if wave==1;

drop yf yf2;

* PROBIT MODEL;

probit yvar $xvars if wave==1;

* Marginal and average effects;
dprobit yvar $xvars if wave==1;

* RESET test;
predict yf, xb;
gen yf2=yf^2;
quietly probit yvar $xvars yf2 if wave==1;
test yf2=0;

drop yf yf2;

* LOGIT MODEL;

logit yvar $xvars if wave==1;

* Marginal and average effects;
mfx compute if e(sample);

* RESET test;
predict yf, xb;
gen yf2=yf^2;
quietly logit yvar $xvars yf2 if wave==1;
test yf2=0;
drop yf yf2;
```

```
********** ORDERED AND MULTINOMIAL CHOICE MODELS *************;

drop yvar;

* ORDERED PROBIT MODEL;

gen yvar=saho;

oprobit yvar $xvars if wave==1, table;
predict yf, xb;
gen yf2=yf^2;
quietly oprobit yvar $xvars yf2 if wave==1;
test yf2=0;
drop yf yf2;
drop yvar;

* BIVARIATE PROBIT MODEL;

gen y1=sah;
gen y2=regfag;

biprobit y1 y2 $xvars if wave==1;

* Marginal and average effects;
mfx compute if e(sample);

drop y1 y2;


********* SELECTION MODEL ****************;

gen yvar=hyfev;

heckman yvar $xvars if wave==1, select($xvars) twostep;
heckman yvar $xvars if wave==1, select($xvars);

drop yvar;


********** COUNT DATA REGRESSION *********;

gen yvar=fagday;

* Poisson model;

poisson yvar $xvars if wave==1;

* Marginal and average effects;
mfx compute if e(sample);

* Negative binomial model;

nbreg yvar $xvars if wave==1;

* Marginal and average effects;
mfx compute if e(sample);
```

```
* Zero inflated negative binomial model;

zinb yvar $xvars if wave==1, inflate(_cons);
zinb yvar $xvars if wave==1, inflate($xvars _cons);


********** PANEL DATA METHODS  *************;

* Random and fixed effects linear regressions;

xtreg yvar $xvars if yvar>0, re i(serno);
xtreg yvar $xvars if yvar>0, fe i(serno);

drop yvar;
gen yvar=sah;

* Pooled probit;

probit yvar $xvars;

*  Marginal and average effects;
dprobit yvar $xvars;

* Random effects probit;

xtprobit yvar $xvars, re i(serno);

* Marginal and average effects;
mfx compute if e(sample), predict(pu0);

* Conditional logit;

xtlogit yvar $xvars, fe i(serno);


log close;
exit;
```

Recent OHE Publications

Consolidation and Competition in the Pharmaceutical Industry
ed. Hannah Kettler, 2001 (price £10.00)

Don't Look Back? Voluntary and Charitable Finance of Hospitals in Britain, Past and Present
by John Mohan and Martin Gorsky, 2001 (price £10.00)

Capturing the Unexpected Benefits of Medical Research
ed. Clive Pritchard, 2001 (price £10.00)

The Economics of the Private Finance Initiative in the NHS
by Jon Sussex, 2001 (price £10.00)

Why Care about Health Inequality?
by Adam Oliver, 2001 (price £7.50)

Health Care Without Frontiers? The Development of a European Market in Health Services?
by Lyndsay Mountford, 2000 (price £10.00)

Productivity Costs: Principles and Practice in Economic Evaluation
by Clive Pritchard and Mark Sculpher, 2000 (price £10.00)

Improving Population Health in Industrialised Nations
ed. Jon Sussex, 2000 (price £10.00)

Surgical Research and Development in the NHS – Promotion, Management and Evaluation
eds. Katharine Johnston and Jon Sussex, 2000 (price £7.50)

The Road to Sustainability in the UK and German Biotechnology Industries
by Hannah Kettler and Steve Casper, 2000 (price £10.00)

Managing to do Better: General Practice in the 21st Century
by Gordon Moore, 2000 (price £7.50)

Prices, Competition and Regulation in Pharmaceuticals: a Cross-national Comparison
by Patricia Danzon and Li-Wei Chao, 2000 (price £10.00)

Benchmarking and Incentives in the NHS
by Paul Grout, Andrew Jenkins and Carol Propper, 2000 (price £7.50)